Practical Ethics in Suicide

Practical Ethics in Suicide

Research, Policy and Clinical Decision-Making

Brian L. Mishara

Université du Québec à Montréal, Canada

David N. Weisstub

International Academy of Law and Mental Health and
Université du Québec à Montréal, Canada

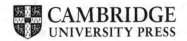

CAMBRIDGE
UNIVERSITY PRESS

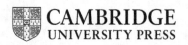

CAMBRIDGE
UNIVERSITY PRESS

Shaftesbury Road, Cambridge CB2 8EA, United Kingdom

One Liberty Plaza, 20th Floor, New York, NY 10006, USA

477 Williamstown Road, Port Melbourne, VIC 3207, Australia

314–321, 3rd Floor, Plot 3, Splendor Forum, Jasola District Centre, New Delhi – 110025, India

103 Penang Road, #05–06/07, Visioncrest Commercial, Singapore 238467

Cambridge University Press is part of Cambridge University Press & Assessment,
a department of the University of Cambridge.

We share the University's mission to contribute to society through the pursuit of
education, learning and research at the highest international levels of excellence.

www.cambridge.org
Information on this title: www.cambridge.org/9781009414906

DOI: 10.1017/9781009414890

© Brian L. Mishara and David N. Weisstub 2024

First published 2024

A catalogue record for this publication is available from the British Library

Library of Congress Cataloging-in-Publication Data
Names: Mishara, Brian L., author. | Weisstub, David N., 1944– author.
Title: Practical ethics in suicide : research, policy and clinical decision
making / Brian L. Mishara, Université du Québec à Montréal, Canada,
David N. Weisstub, International Academy of Law and Mental Health.
Description: Cambridge, United Kingdom ; New York, NY, USA : Cambridge
University Press, 2024. | Includes bibliographical references and index.
Identifiers: LCCN 2023041805 | ISBN 9781009414906 (paperback) | ISBN
9781009414890 (ebook)
Subjects: LCSH: Suicide – Moral and ethical aspects. | Suicide – Social
aspects. | Suicide – Psychological aspects. | Suicide – Prevention. |
Assisted suicide – Moral and ethical aspects.
Classification: LCC HV6545 .M517 2024 | DDC 362.28–dc23/eng/20231117
LC record available at https://lccn.loc.gov/2023041805

ISBN 978-1-009-41490-6 Paperback

Contents

Preface

Suicide is a major health problem worldwide. According to World Health Organization (WHO) data, almost 700,000 people die by suicide each year (World Health Organization, 2021a). There are more deaths by suicide annually than in all wars, conflicts, terrorist acts, and homicides combined. Surprisingly, there are fewer research studies on suicide than on many less common causes of mortality. This is at least in part because ethical considerations lead to limitations on the nature of research investigations on the subject. The first part of this book examines specific ethical issues concerning suicide research, policies, and practices. The latter chapters focus on the ethical and legal quandaries surrounding another intentional means of ending one's life, Medical Assistance in Dying (MAiD), which includes the practices of euthanasia and assisted suicide.

The issues are explored through case studies and examples, including: the role of telephone helplines and internet assistance, questions surrounding identifying a genetic basis for suicidal behaviour, the historical precedents of mental illness treatments, and specific legal and ethical approaches to MAiD.

Ethical perspectives are presented on the acceptability of suicidal behaviours and the obligations and limitations of intervening to prevent suicides. In suicide interventions, lives are potentially at stake. For this reason, intervention protocols must clarify if extreme measures are to be undertaken to save a life, and we must decide whether research protocols should be held to a higher standard than for studies of less consequential matters. Ethical concerns may influence whether or not potentially life-saving interventions will be undertaken, and under which circumstances, as well as what is permissible in research studies. It is our premise that the resolution of ethical issues concerning suicide is not based upon straightforward applications of general ethical principles or guidelines. Both explicit and implicit moral and ethical beliefs that may vary depending upon the circumstances inevitably influence decisions we make.

The issue of MAiD, the Canadian label for the practices of active euthanasia and assisted suicide, is often designated as posing ethical challenges that are different from the issues concerning suicide prevention. Both MAiD and suicide involve an intentional decision to die prematurely. We demonstrate that there is substantial overlap in the ethical implications of these two domains, which we analyse in several chapters in this volume.

Articulation of clear moral premises is essential in determining how common ethical issues concerning suicide may be resolved. In general, we do not promote a specific moral position but believe that it is useful to explore implicit moral premises and their ethical bases in order to understand current practices and to decide upon future policies and courses of action. However, on several issues, we expose a penchant towards reserving death as a solution of last resort. Before examining specific ethical dilemmas, we describe several paradigmatic positions concerning suicide in Chapter 1, in order to facilitate analyses of ethical issues that arise in diverse contexts.

Suicide has been topical since ancient times, whether in the Judaeo-Christian tradition of theological commentaries, or in the hands of preeminent philosophers who considered suicide a subject worthy of contemplation. In these traditions, a wealth of material has emerged over the centuries that has directed our attention to where to place suicide, whether it should be perceived as an elevated act of ending life to achieve a memorial of reaching to the clouds, or as a tragic act of dejection, defeat, and misery. Celebrated philosophical analyses have been the subject of public debates and more recently have been witnessed by larger and larger groups through social media, journalism, and town hall discussions, often of a highly vocal nature. In a certain sense, intentionally ending life by suicide or MAiD has become central to the questions about the type of society that we wish to support: For example: How much credit do we wish to give to individual decision-making, even when the individual is handicapped mentally or physically? What are the limits of respect to be given to professionals arriving out of the elite bodies of law and medicine?

This book concerns people who may be faced with difficult decisions about life and death, most of whom have not been schooled in the illustrious debates of prior centuries. We can ask what value there is in philosophising for hands-on practitioners who function in a Good-Samaritan role. What are the consequences of simplifying nuanced philosophical standpoints and applying them to the world of practitioners? It is our view that an examination of our ethical premises and alternative perspectives can help clarify the morally grey areas that present themselves in suicide prevention.

The positions we present in this volume should be regarded as a starting point, meant to stimulate discussion. This book aims to encourage people who have committed their lives to suicide prevention and research to engage in discussions and debate, to help better understand the moral implications of decisions that they, our institutions, and our societies are making.

Acknowledgements

We thank Steven Stack, Nancy Logue, and Terry Carney for their insightful comments on earlier versions of this book, Luc Dargis for his diligent work in verifying the bibliography, Steve Carriere and Sara Derbel for administrative support, Catherine Goulet-Cloutier for secretarial help, Anh Tu Tran for verifying country laws concerning suicide, and the CRISE research centre members and colleagues whose collaboration is greatly appreciated.

1

· · · · · · ·

Ethical Perspectives
to Guide Decision-Making

Should the lives of suicidal people be saved whenever possible? The answer to that question has been debated by philosophers and policymakers since humanity's earliest historical records. Today, we find the standard range of philosophical orientations revealed in contemporary practices and bioethical discussions. The general ethical perspectives presented in this chapter are succinct statements of alternative positions one may take concerning the moral acceptability or unacceptability of suicide, as well as one's obligations to intervene to save a life and the limits thereof. Our presentation of philosophical perspectives is intentionally abbreviated, sidestepping many subtleties of the rich debates among philosophers on these issues. However, we use this overview to set out a framework for thinking about the implicit and explicit ethical premises that underlie existing policies and practices concerning suicide and suicide prevention. We present popular paradigms or conventional models of the ethics of suicide research culture to articulate how these points of view may make a difference in applied situations. Although, in our view, pure philosophical forms are unlikely to be found in real-life moral dilemmas, we think it may be genuinely beneficial for practitioners, researchers, and policymakers to acknowledge and communicate their own values and how these values inform the resolution of hard cases in suicide research ethics (Stojanović, 2020; Weisstub, 1998).

Attitudes towards the acceptability of suicide vary around the world, and individuals within countries hold a variety of beliefs about whether suicide is justified. The seventh World Values Survey, completed in 2021 (Haerpfer *et al.*, 2022), includes data from a survey from 80 countries, with 1,000 to 5,000 respondents per country. Participants were asked, as part of a detailed questionnaire about their values, 'Please tell me whether you think suicide can always be justified, never be justified, or somewhere in between?' Respondents were given a card with a scale from 1, labelled 'never justified', to 10, labelled 'always justified', to indicate their response. Overall, countries having more secular-rational values that place less emphasis on religion, traditional family values, and authority are more accepting of suicide, although they do not necessarily have more suicides, when compared with countries with more traditional values. The mean scores, on the scale from 1 to 10 (1 = never justified; 10 = always justified) vary from 1.12 for Egypt to 5.21 for the Netherlands.

Some countries, such as Egypt and Albania, have almost universal beliefs that suicide is never acceptable (in Egypt 95.3% of respondents answered 1; in Albania 93.9%). This contrasts with countries where most people held a middle view, with relatively few feeling that suicide is never acceptable (e.g., in the Netherlands 15% responded 'never acceptable' and 11.4% 'always acceptable'). In analyses of Wave 4 of the World Values Surveys (1999–2001), Stack and Kposowa (2016) found that cultural approval of suicide was associated with values of individual self-expression. These data indicate that although there are significant differences in how much people feel suicide is justifiable by country, we see a range of beliefs *within* all countries, and in most countries the majority feel that some suicides are justified.

We have identified three broadly defined positions, recurrent in discourses concerning suicide, which we call moralist, libertarian, and relativist. These positions express the dominant perspectives that are the usual starting points for how both experts and laypeople orient themselves in problematic or conflictual situations. This chapter is meant to suggest possible opening conversations, ways of looking that should lead us in the quest for greater dialogue.

1.1 In the Name of Morality

Several philosophical traditions adhere to the moralist position that suicide is unacceptable and that there is a pervasive moral obligation to protect life. Arguments against the acceptability of suicide have a long history
in several different philosophical traditions. They may be based upon a
religious philosophy in which it is sinful to take one's own life, such as is
clearly indicated in the Koran. The teachings of Mohammed require sub-
mitting to divine will and one's preordained destiny (Kismet), which includes the timing of death. The Koran states that suicide is a graver crime
than homicide: 'O believers! ... do not kill ⌐each other or⌐ yourselves. Surely
Allah is ever Merciful to you [...] And whoever does this sinfully and un-
justly, We will burn them in the Fire. That is easy for Allah' (Khattab, 2016,
4:29, 4:30)

The concept that suicide goes against divine law and is unacceptable can
be found first in the views of the pre-Socratic philosopher Pythagoras who,
according to Plato's accounts, believed that people must wait until God re-
leases the soul from its bonds, despite the ordeals of living (Choron, 1972;
Stojanović, 2020). Plato concurred that suicide is disgraceful and wrote
that suicides should be buried ignominiously in unmarked graves (Plato,
1934). However, Plato recognised that there are some exceptions: when
one's mind is morally corrupted, when the self-killing is done by judicial
order, when the suicide is compelled by extreme unavoidable misfortunes,
and when it is from shame after having committed grossly unjust actions.

Although there is no prohibition against suicide in Christian scriptures,
and suicides by martyrdom were admired in early Christian writings, the
status of suicide as a crime and sin was incorporated into Christian dogma
beginning with St Augustine in the fourth century (Dublin and Bunzel,
1933), who considered suicide to be an unrepentable sin. By the time
of Thomas Aquinas in the thirteenth century, suicide was recognised as
both a sin and a crime. His arguments that life itself is sacred, that suicide
disrespects the authority and generosity of the Creator, and that suicide
leaves no opportunity for repentance have remained a fundamental part
of Christian doctrines (Barrois, 1945).

Moralist arguments against the acceptability of suicide need not be based upon religious or social obligations; for example, they can include a justification based on the categorical imperative of Immanuel Kant (1949). Kant believed that human life is sacred and must be preserved at all costs, as part of moral law that dictates this obligation categorically and unconditionally. He wrote in *The Metaphysics of Morals*, 'The preservation of one's own life ... is a duty', and 'To dispose of one's life for some fancied end is to degrade the humanity subsisting in his person and entrusted to him to the end that he might uphold and preserve it' (Kant, 1949, p. 239). Although Kant believed in the duty to preserve life, he was concerned about some exceptional circumstances when he questioned if a heroic death to save one's country should be considered a suicide, and whether it is a suicide if a person condemned to die is commanded to kill himself (as Nero commanded Seneca). Kant also asked if it is a suicide when a person bitten by a rabid dog, knowing he will die from the wound, kills himself to avoid endangering others. As Jacques Choron (1972) points out, these questions are more than attempts to define what is a suicide and what is not. They reflect potential challenges to Kant's main contention that for moral reasons suicide is unacceptable, without offering answers or revising his strong commitment to his belief in preserving life.

The moralist position is that the protection of life is a fundamental value that takes precedence in decision-making. Other theological arguments include the necessity to conform to God's intentions, leaving it to the Creator to determine the timing and manner of death. One can also find arguments condemning suicide based on natural law, including St Thomas' contention that suicide is contrary to natural inclinations to charity, whereby every man should love himself.

Arguments that date back to Aristotle contend that suicide harms other people and the society in which one lives. An individual has the responsibility to remain alive and serve society and not be cowardly and kill oneself to escape 'from poverty or love or anything painful' (Aristotle, 2000, 1116.10). This view of suicide as a harm to society has been expressed in various ways over time. For example, in sixteenth-century England, suicide was viewed as an offence against the King's interest in the preservation of all his subjects, albeit based on their economic value as taxpayers. Obligations towards society are also reflected in the contemporary argument that taking one's life has disastrous effects on the person's family and friends.

This harm to society is sometimes the basis for laws that make suicide illegal (see Chapter 7). Most countries have decriminalised suicidal behaviours, though a minority still maintain its illegality. For example, Canada decriminalised suicide in 1972 (Lester, 1992), and England in 1961 (England, 1961). Most Western countries have laws against aiding and abetting suicides. Chapter 7 reviews the legal status of suicide around the world and looks at the arguments for and against laws criminalising suicide.

Regardless of the justifications given, the moralist position is that it is essential to save and preserve life in all circumstances, and that suicide prevention is an imperative.

1.2   Self-Styled Libertarianism

Libertarian perspectives emphasise the individual's freedom of choice to determine whether to live or die. Libertarian perspectives vary in their philosophical basis, from the hedonistic right to suicide to avoid pain to a wide range of utilitarian approaches. For example, Hume (1894) insisted that not a single text of Scripture prohibits suicide and said that the commandment 'Thou shalt not kill' is meant to only exclude the killing of others. He argued that when people experience pain and suffering, and when a person is tired of life and is more a burden than an asset, suicide can be the prudent and courageous way to react to misfortune.

Libertarian views of suicide may be found in contemporary beliefs that the decision to live and die may be weighed rationally by a contemplative individual who is not currently suffering (Nashnoush and Sheikh, 2021; Prado, 1998). A more radical libertarian approach involves actively promoting suicide under certain circumstances; for example, for those suffering from a painful or debilitating physical illness (Humphry, 1991; Nashnoush and Sheikh, 2021). Regardless of whether the justification for a libertarian perspective concerns an obligation to avoid pain and displeasure or a simple neutrality with respect to life-and-death decisions, the net result is that from a libertarian point of view there is no specific obligation to intervene to prevent a suicide.

The trend towards a more libertarian perspective on suicide may be reflected in the decriminalisation of suicidal behaviours in many countries. For some, the practices of euthanasia and assisted suicide constitute an embodiment of this perspective, and the legalisation of these practices in some countries indicates their increasing influence. However, it is important to note that those who are proponents of euthanasia often distinguish between end-of-life decisions by the terminally ill and persons with incurable degenerative diseases, and suicidal behaviour by persons suffering from mental illness (Humphry, 1991; Nicolini *et al.*, 2020). The libertarian perspective is that such distinctions, requiring special precautions, need not be made public policy nor guide clinical interventions and research on suicide. As existential philosophers have contended, libertarian perspectives recognise an inherent 'right' to decide whether life is worth living (Camus, 1955), and the absence of an obligation to interfere with the personal decision to die.

1.3   The Umbrella of Relativism

In ethical philosophy, *relativism* refers to the belief that what is morally acceptable varies according to the context or framework of assessment. That framework may be local cultural or contextual norms or individual standards (Baghramian and Carter, 2022). Relativist perspectives (Macklin, 1999; Mishara and Weisstub, 2018) determine the 'rightness' or 'wrongness' of suicide, and the extent to which there are obligations to intervene to prevent suicide, based upon either contemporary situational and cultural variables or on the anticipated consequences of action or inaction. A large proportion of the general public may be considered common-sense contextualists since they reply differently to questions about the acceptability of suicide depending upon the nature of the situation. For example, people in many cultures generally feel the suicide of an elderly person to be more acceptable than the suicide of a young person; suicide is generally more accepted if the person is suffering from a painful terminal illness than if the person is healthy.

Different ethical and religious groups may hold opposing views about which suicides should be condemned and which should be condoned or accepted. However, from the relativist perspective, the specific context and consequences matter for determining the morality. For example, the Stoics in ancient Greece are noted for their acceptance of suicide. The virtues of suicide were praised by Seneca for elders who begin to lose their faculties and by Pliny the Younger, who considered suicide to be 'eminently high and praiseworthy'. Nevertheless, the Stoics had a contextualist view in which not all suicides were acceptable. Noble suicides that resulted from careful deliberation were accepted or praised. However, impulsive suicides, due to temporary 'confusion of values', or ones done in the absence of sufficient cause were clearly unacceptable. For example, Epictetus said,

> But remember the principal thing: that the door is open.
> Do not be more fearful than children; but as they, when the
> play doth not please them, say, 'I will play no longer':
> so do you, in the same case, say, 'I will play no longer', and go;
> but, if you stay, do not complain.
>
> (Epictetus, 1910, p. 49)

The Stoics accepted suicides resulting from careful deliberation in unendurable circumstances but rejected rash suicides and suicides in more tolerable situations. This contrasts with Jewish laws, as formulated in the Mishnah of the Talmud, which stipulated that, 'Whenever a person of sane mind destroys his own life, he shall not be bothered with at all.' The Talmudic commentary by Rabbi Eleazar summarises the funeral practises: 'Leave him in the clothes in which he died, honour him not, nor damn him. One does not tear his garments on his account, nor take off one's shoes, nor does one hold funeral rites for him; but one does comfort the family, for that is honouring the living' (Preuss, 1911, pp. 603–607). In the Semachot, a post-Talmudic treatise on the rules of mourning, Chapter 2 discusses when a person found dead should be regarded as a suicide, or 'one who intentionally destroys himself' ('*meabed atzmo ladaat*').

In the case of suicide (intentional self-destruction), the Semachot indicates that the person's body is deprived of all ritual honours. However, the definition of suicide requires that the act was with full intention ('*ladaat*'). This requirement and the Talmudic requirement that the person be of 'sound mind' indicate that suicides resulting from rational deliberation, which were accepted and in some circumstances encouraged by the Stoics, are the only acts of self-destruction that are condemned in traditional Jewish practices. Jewish practice does not consider a death to be a suicide if the person's intentions were not 'full' or if the person was not of sound mind. This would eliminate most deaths classified as suicide by coroners and medical examiners. Up to 90% of people who die by suicide in Western countries, and at least a majority elsewhere (Cho *et al.*, 2016; Knipe *et al.*, 2019), have a diagnosable mental disorder, so they could be considered to potentially not be of 'sound mind.'

The view that the determination of a death as a suicide in Jewish practice should be limited is further supported by analyses of the meaning of the Hebrew word '*ladaat*' and its practical implications. Perls (1911) stated that the full intention to end one's life must have been clearly expressed in words before the death. For example, if a person is found hanging on a tree or pierced by his own sword, this is not considered a suicide, because it could have been a murder if the person had not announced his plan to kill himself beforehand. Friedlander (1915, p. 213) quoted the Orthodox Jewish laws pertaining to suicide, which include:

> When one who had been killed was discovered, as far as possible the act of killing should be regarded as the deed of another person and not as his own deed. If a child dies by suicide, it is considered that he

had done the deed unwittingly. Likewise, if an adult killed himself and it is evident that the act was prompted by madness or through fear of terrible torture, he should be treated as an ordinary deceased person.

Although it may appear that Orthodox Jewish practices express an absolutist position in which all suicides are unacceptable, the acceptance of killing oneself in justifiable circumstances (madness, fear of torture, when a child, without clearly expressed full intentions) indicates that the position can arguably be described as contextualist, notwithstanding that exceptions do not necessarily nullify a guiding principle.

Furthermore, ambivalence about suicide in suicidal individuals has been found to be omnipresent by many researchers (Macintyre *et al.*, 2021). Given that a high proportion of people who kill themselves are suffering from a mental disorder and are considered to have ambivalent feelings, only the very few people who kill themselves in a rational, unequivocal, and deliberate manner would meet the Jewish definition of suicide.

Another relativist perspective, based upon a utilitarian ethic, focuses on the best interests of society as understood in terms of the cost–benefit analysis of social utility, rather than just on the best interests of the person. Underlying the utilitarian ethic is the maximisation of social utility as the vehicle to alleviate social misery. For the utilitarian, suicide sometimes may be viewed as an honourable behaviour that preserves and respects societal values, for example in the case of hara-kiri and kamikaze deaths in Japan. In other contexts, for example in the former Soviet Republics, suicide was viewed negatively because it deprived society of the productivity of a worker. Therefore, suicide was regarded as an aggression against state interests, as was the case earlier in feudal England.

All the diverse relativist perspectives share the common view that the obligation to protect life varies, depending upon an analysis of the context or situation. The analysis may be in terms of an understanding of the cultural context and current circumstances, or an assessment of the consequences for the person, their milieu, or society. Such reflection may involve some form of cost–benefit (or risk–advantage) analysis of the situation, based on principles ranging from individualist to communitarian values.

1.4   The Rationality of Suicide

The philosopher Jacques Choron (1964) defined *rational suicide* as meeting the following criteria: (1) there is no psychiatric disorder; (2) there is no impairment of reasoning; and (3) the person's motives appear to be justifiable or at least understandable by the majority of contemporaries in the same culture or social group. Choron's first requirement, that there is no psychiatric disorder, eliminates the majority of suicides, since most people who die by suicide suffer from a mental disorder. This indicates that rational suicide, if it exists, characterises only a small minority of suicides (Knoll IV, 2019; Prado, 2008).

Even the most vocal proponents of the possible rationality of suicide exclude people suffering from mental disorders. Humphry (1986), in his defence of the Hemlock Society's support of rational suicide, states that there is another form, 'emotional suicide or irrational self-murder'. The Hemlock Society's stance or policy on nonrational suicide is to prevent it whenever possible. Furthermore, the Society explicitly discouraged any form of suicide 'for mental health or unhappy reasons' (Humphry, 1986). In recent years, this narrow support for rational suicide has been expanded to include those persons whose suffering is emotional and is associated with the presence of a mental disorder (see Chapter 8).

When the person who attempts suicide does not suffer from a serious mental disorder, suicide may still be irrational; for example, when a person is in a temporary state of extreme agitation or emotional despair. When a person has suffered a loss, been abandoned by a spouse, or been fired from a job, they may become highly suicidal even though they have not been suffering from a previous mental disorder.

There remains the question of whether any suicide can be considered rational. Ron Maris (1982) argued that suicide derives from one's inability or refusal to accept the terms of the human condition. He felt that suicide may be seen as effectively solving the problems at hand, in contrast to nonsuicidal alternatives. In his view, although no suicide is ever the best alternative to our common human condition, for some individuals suicide expresses a logical response to an existential human situation.

The philosopher Margaret Battin (1984), while admitting that no human acts are ever wholly rational, defines 'rational suicide' in terms of the criteria of the person being able to reason, having a realistic world view, possessing adequate information, and acting in accordance with their own fundamental interests. Battin indicates that meeting the criterion of 'the ability to reason' appears to be very difficult, as research and anecdotal information indicate that people who die by suicide often leave messages that are illogical and tend to refer to themselves as being able to perceive the effects of their suicide after their own death. One of the basic criteria for being able to act rationally is the ability to use logical processes and to see the causal consequences of one's actions. It can be argued that the majority of suicidal persons do not accurately foresee consequences.

In addition, one can pose the philosophical question of whether it is possible to foresee the final consequence of suicide, which constitutes knowing what it is like to be dead. Battin suggests that when we imagine ourselves dead, we generally project ourselves as viewing our own dead body surrounded by grieving relatives at a gravesite. This presupposes a subject with a specific capacity. Battin acknowledges two classes of suicides that are not necessarily irrational. First are those with religious or metaphysical beliefs that include the possibility that one goes on to have human-like experiences after death. Second are persons whose reputation and honour are of primary importance (e.g., a Japanese suicide of honour) or collective suicides aimed to protect the dignity of a specific group (e.g., the mass suicide of the Jews at Masada).

There is also the challenging question of what constitutes rational decision-making. Rationality, according to *Webster's New World Dictionary of the American Language* (1966), is 'exercising one's reason in a proper manner, having sound judgment; sensible, sane; not foolish, absurd or extravagant; implying the ability to reason logically, as by drawing conclusions from inferences, and often connoting the absence of emotion' (p. 1207).

This definition implies a degree of autonomy in the decision-making process, the ability to engage in logical and reasoned thought processes, and the absence of undue influence on the decision-making process by external factors. Professor David Mayo (1983), in a review of contemporary philosophical writings on suicide, suggests that a rational suicide must realistically consider alternatives with the likelihood of realising goals of fundamental interest to the person. The person then must choose an alternative that will maximise the realisation of those goals. Mishara (1998) has argued that most important human decision-making is more emotional than rational, including significant choices in life, such as whom we marry and what careers we choose. If important decisions have a predominantly emotional basis, what would lead one to expect that the paramount decision of ending one's life could be different and more rational? Those who argue for the existence of rational suicide (e.g., Benatar, 2020) generally insist that this must occur when a person is experiencing interminable suffering. Mishara argues that in the presence of severe suffering, true rational decision-making is even less likely to occur; the emotions associated with the suffering compromise one's ability to think rationally.

Battin addresses the criteria for rational decision-making in terms of the decision being based on a realistic view of the world. She points out that there are multiple world views, which vary depending on cultural and religious beliefs; what appears to be irrational for some is considered quite rational in other cultural contexts. Her third criterion, that the person possesses adequate information, may need to be reframed to consider the impact of the emotional state of the person on their ability to evaluate and consider information, and, by implication, to be able to consider alternative courses of action. The vast majority of suicides occur at critical junctures of the life cycle.

Battin's additional criterion of avoidance of harm is essentially the justification that organisations such as the Hemlock Society propose as their fundamental justification for rational suicide. They cite the cessation of the harm caused by unbearable suffering as the most common reason for suicide. They reference grave physical handicap, which can be so constricting or extreme that the individual finds it intolerable. This justification goes against Christian and other religious traditions that view pain and suffering as serving the constructive purpose of spiritual growth, having a deeper meaning, or as being part of God's plan.

The decision to end one's life when terminally ill is frequently represented as the most rational basis for suicide. The acceptance of ending life when extreme pain or handicap is experienced assumes that no relief for the pain is available and that the severe handicap cannot be tolerated. Humphry (1986) defends people's 'right' to refuse to experience even a 'beneficent lingering' and to simply choose to discontinue living when terminally ill.

Battin's (1984) final criterion, 'acting in accordance with a person's fundamental interest', raises the question of whether one can actually satisfy personal interest by being dead (and not around to be satisfied). Nevertheless, some individuals have long-standing moral beliefs in which the decision to shorten life under difficult circumstances is condoned as being 'in their interest'.

The concept of rational suicide may be confused with the concept of 'understandable' suicide. The psychologist David Clarke (1999) suggests that, when considering the expressed wish to die, the concepts of rationality and autonomy are less useful than the concepts of 'understandability' and 'respect'. It is essential to point out, however, that what an outsider might consider to be understandable or respectful of a person's wishes is often not symmetrical with the suicidal person's experience. In some situations, when outsiders feel that a person would be 'better off dead', those who are existentially grounded in a harsh reality feel differently. Despite popular belief, very few persons who are suffering from terminal and severely disabling chronic illnesses seriously consider, or engage in, behaviour to end life prematurely (Choy, 2017; Liu *et al.*, 2020; Mishara, 1998, 1999b).

Debates concerning rational suicide often centre around society's obligations to provide easier access to suicide under specified conditions, implying moral acceptance. The haunting question remains where and how to assess the requisite threshold of rationality. What constitutes unbearable suffering for one person may be an acceptable level of discomfort for another. Furthermore, individuals differ in the extent to which rationality is the key component of their decision-making processes. On what basis may we say that rational decision-making is more justifiable than emotionally driven decisions? Most suicidologists choose to try to prevent suicides that come to their attention, assuming that rational suicides, if they exist, are rare; that they are difficult to identify; and, finally, that they merit interventions to challenge their reasoning.

1.5   The Rational Obligation to Suicide

Some have argued that there are circumstances when there can be a rational obligation to suicide, a duty to suicide. The philosopher Joel Feinberg defined a duty as something required of one to be done whether we like it or not (Feinberg, 1980). A moral duty may be associated with a larger community, where sanctions may be attached in the event of failing to act morally.

Immanuel Kant is often viewed as the preeminent philosopher of deontology (the study of duty or moral obligation), and his absolutist stance against suicide is widely known. However, some Kantian scholars have identified various exceptions to this view and have made arguments in favour of a duty to commit suicide under certain conditions. Despite ongoing debates about the proper interpretation of Kant on this matter, Altman (2020), a Kant scholar, argues that the positions taken by interpreters who claim that Kant provides an inroad for an obligation to die are a serious misinterpretation of his work as a whole.

These 'interpreters' claim that Kant believed that a person who has lost her moral agency should view suicide not only sympathetically, but also as a duty. They argue that this approach is based on the principle that the moral must trump the physical, and when a person is no longer able to act morally, the protection of life should be suspended. Kant himself referenced the case of a galley slave who had lost the capacity to act as an agent in his own right, likening him to an animal. This understanding of the loss of moral agency has been developed by scholars such as Dennis Cooley

(2015a, 2015b) and James Callahan (1995), who argue for a duty to suicide, subject to certain conditions.

Cooley criticised Kant's position, identifying what he contends is a serious shortcoming in what he calls 'moral psychology'. He argues for the establishment of duty to suicide when moral agency is no longer present. It is worth noting that in situations of extreme scarcity of resources, deadly conflicts, torture, starvation, and complete degradation of self, it may be difficult to determine what constitutes moral agency.

From our perspective it is difficult to assert that lack of moral agency remains the correct characterisation when there is scarcity of resources, or when deadly conflicts have resulted in torture, starvation, and complete degradation of self. Shall we include the particular vulnerabilities of women who have been disallowed from moral agency in some theocratic cultures?

The problem with fashioning moral agency is that the exceptions give rise to a more fundamental question of who could possibly be the rightful judge of what constitutes moral agency in the face of calamitous conditions. There is a danger in citing abstract health-care situations that suit a philosophical argument for lack of moral agency. Survivors of atrocities have confronted the profound loss of moral agency in different ways: for example, finding meaning in life despite their circumstances, surviving to bear witness, and honouring fallen parents through the propagation of future generations. Moral agency alone is not the informative characterisation of action when unspeakable acts result in a diffusion of self.

In considering the social welfare medicine found in Western Europe and many Commonwealth countries, there are still many inconsistencies in who pays for what, and whether such inequalities are conducive to the wealthy having a greater, better, or more credible moral agency in contrast to vulnerable minorities, women, children and adolescents, and the impoverished. End-of-life costs are massive, and there can be compelling reasons for ending life found in the many narratives of retaining funds for loved ones.

Dennis Cooley presented the case of the Canadian Gillian Bennett, who died in August 2014 by suicide to avoid succumbing to dementia (Cooley, 2015b). Bennett's video diary, which has been watched worldwide, demonstrated an apparently thoughtful and dignified approach to her own death. Recognising how a decreased mental capacity would alter her agency, and expressing her thankfulness to her next of kin, Bennett disclaimed any remorse in embracing death. Cooley cited her as a role model. Her life was a special one, with a loving relationship with her husband and her extended family. She was the beneficiary of an enlightened social welfare medical community. Given her heightened sense of not being a burden to her family, she also conveyed a sense of responsibility to her country for the good life that she had lived.

To what extent was Gillian Bennett's suicide a model to be followed? Kant's proclamation, 'To live is not a necessity; but to live honourably while life lasts is a necessity' (Kant, 1963, p. 152), is a general statement that may not apply to every individual or situation, particularly those who are less fortunate. One can imagine the reaction of powerful, autocratic, and dictatorial cultures that could mock and humiliate people who are thought to lack the dignity to take their own lives under predetermined circumstances. In our view, this would be the ultimate distortion of what Kant and his many interpreters intended.

The relevance of the body as deteriorations occur is also a complex issue. It is important to ensure that individuals with physical or mental handicaps are not discriminated against or devalued, and that their lives are considered just as valuable as anyone else's. As we discuss in more detail in Chapter 8, in their vehement condemnation of the Canadian expansion of the MAiD laws to include persons with degenerative handicaps and mental illness, organisations and individuals with physical disabilities have expressed that the use of a physical or mental handicap as a criterion for euthanasia and assisted suicide is prejudicial and constitutes a fundamental devaluation of the lives of people who are entitled to the supports necessary to live a fulfilling life (United Nation Human Rights Committee (HRC), 3 September 2019; United Nation Human Rights Council, 26 September 2019; Commission spéciale sur la question de mourir dans la dignité, 2012; Vulnerable Persons Secretariat, 2020). In 2019, the UNHRC Special Rapporteur on the Rights of Persons with Disabilities reported that she was told by persons with disabilities that they were offered the illusory 'choice' between living in a nursing home and having their lives ended by MAiD (Devandas-Aguilar and United Nation Human Rights Council Special Rapporteur on the Rights of Persons with Disabilities, December 19, 2019). The Special Rapporteur and the Independent Expert on the enjoyment of human rights by older persons sent a joint communication to Canada (Quinn *et al.*, 2021) in which they expressed concerns that the Canadian MAiD laws discriminate against the elderly and persons with disabilities by viewing their lives as being of lesser value, a form of prejudice they referred to as 'ableism'.

There is no consensus about who is the rightful person to intercede in clarifying options or supposed duties. In such situations we find ourselves in a quagmire of moral confusion. Even when individuals and their families have agreed that they have become a burden, there will be examples of unsustainable guilt at having allowed a suicide of kin to go forward. Given the scarcity of resources and the projection that increasing numbers of people will be called upon to assist those in a diminished state, can we foresee a society that will be bent on preparing citizens to release their guilt in favour of dutiful suicides?

And what of the unequal pressure on the dispossessed, which reinforces their lower social status and asserts their lesser worth? Should this lead to a particular course of action, an affirmation, or a clear denial of the duty to suicide because of their historical and present dispossession? Rosemary Tong (2000) noted that because women are more nurturing and self-sacrificing than men, the concept of a duty to die might be unreasonably applied to them. This argument can be equally applied to minority communities where there are conflictual senses of obligation.

Bioethicists such as Dena Davis (2015) have asserted that to seize control of one's destiny, especially under circumstances of great tragedy and limits, is to be active and dominant. This incites women to take charge of their lives as full persons with moral obligations to fulfil. Although this is a statement of principle that resounds morally, its practical applicability across countries remains perplexing due to global inequities.

In this regard it is instructive to return to Kant's treatment of Lucretia's historic suicide, which altered the direction of the Roman Empire. Kant wrote:

> The moment I can no longer live in honour but become unworthy by such an action, I can no longer live at all ... if, for instance, a woman cannot preserve her life any longer except by surrendering her person to the will of another, she is bound to give up her life rather than dishonour humanity in her own person. (Kant, 1963, p. 156)

Can anyone today credibly make such a moral claim as a protocol for women who are raped? Many would find Kant's statement morally repulsive. Is this yet another form of victim-blaming cast as agency? It is illuminating to reflect on the Kantian view that an individual should first resist rather than take their own life. Again, Kant's comments may be considered a philosopher's luxury and ignorant of the reality in which victims find themselves.

Once euthanasia is legalised and medically assisted dying is put into place in a jurisdiction, what implications are there for the expanding territory of a duty to die? There are sets of criteria that have been offered to assist us in making informed decisions personally or societally about the duty to suicide. Hardwig's suggested criteria for a duty to die are one example:

1. Continuing to live will impose significant burdens on your family and loved ones as you grow older.
2. If you have lived a full and rich life.
3. If your loved ones' lives have already been difficult or impoverished.
4. If your loved ones have made great contributions to make your life a great one.
5. If you cannot make a good adjustment to your illness.
6. If you cannot make significant contributions to others, especially your family.
7. If the part of you that is loved will soon be gone or seriously compromised.

8. If you have lived a relatively lavish lifestyle instead of saving for your illness or old age. (Hardwig, 1997a, 1997b)

Nothing of the aforementioned criteria is written in stone or is compelling as a firm guideline. Culture, gender, religion, and other factors could suggest other criteria or none at all. Whatever the criteria, there are concerns about manipulating and exploiting the vulnerable.

In his unpacking of Kant's deficiencies in the area of 'moral psychology', Cooley (2013) quoted the work of Virginia Held (1996, p. 36)

> This is not to say that rationality should be abandoned; it is to say that rationality must be tried out in and revised in the light of moral experience and must be supplemented by the moral understanding that can only be cultivated by embodied, empathic actual persons.

In looking back to the Bennett diary, the compelling question is whether it expressed a duty to die or more simply was a statement about a life no longer seeming to be worth living, where 'duty' does not really describe her state of mind and her message to the world.

Once we enter a wider world where we are concerned about the manipulation of vulnerable populations, the real crux of the matter is exposed. Most individuals are neither noblemen nor philosophers. They are subject to deteriorations of self and handicaps, both physical and mental, more often present at the end stages of life. It is possible that, with population growth and the elderly living to breakthrough ages, withdrawal of support will become a threat to the incapacitated and dying. We need to be ready morally to answer arguments about the duty to die.

Are we doomed to passively venture towards alleviating guilt and accepting that citizens must plan to terminate themselves at an appropriate time consonant with a new morality? It is premature to celebrate such a duty. In fact, at this stage in our contemporary life it would be widely regarded as a deplorable move. Perhaps Kant's notion of moral agency is 'so reasoned through' with an array of interpretations that it is eclipsed by the realities of death and family in an age of scarcity and growth in inequalities.

In the future, technologies and medical innovations may develop to compensate for what we know as handicaps. What appears now as an utterly hopeless future could become a tolerable reality. In the latter part of the twentieth century a diagnosis of active acquired immunodeficiency syndrome (AIDS) was considered a death sentence accompanied by decreasing capacity, increased suffering and dependency, and an apparent loss of personhood. Suicide rates among people with AIDS increased dramatically, particularly suicide among persons when first diagnosed with human immunodeficiency virus (HIV), before serious symptoms appeared. Medical advances have now resulted in people with AIDS being able to live fulfilling lives. It is possible that in a relatively short period of time other afflictions that have been described as warranting a duty to die may be alleviated or sufficiently diminished.

1.6   The Right to Be Protected from Committing Suicide

Jonathan Herring (2022) has argued that suicidal individuals have a basic right in the United Kingdom (UK) to receive treatment and have actions taken to protect them from killing themselves. Citing various court decisions, he contends that every vulnerable person must be protected from death. For example, in the case of *Rabone* (*Rabone and another* (*Appellants*) *v Pennine Care NHS Trust* (*Respondent*) [2012]) Lady Justice Hale, herself an expert in mental health law, opined that there should be laws to deal with 'threats to life from any quarter' (Hale *et al.*, 2017).

Professor Herring cites the European Convention on Human Rights (ECHR), Article 2 (the Right to Life) as the justification for providing protection of life by suicide prevention activities, citing *Olewnik-Cieplińska and Olewnik v. Poland* [2019]:

> However, the scope of the positive obligation must be interpreted in a way which does not impose an impossible or disproportionate burden on the authorities. Not every claimed risk to life, therefore,

can entail for the authorities a convention requirement to take operational measures to prevent that risk from materialising.

This judgement indicates that the obligation to protect from suicide risk is tempered by what is practical, and it can depend upon an analysis of how burdensome it is to respond to a potential need for protection. To date, the right to be protected from suicide has not been included in any specific legislation, and judges in the UK and elsewhere have been reluctant to insist that any specific suicide prevention actions must be undertaken. At best, as judges have said, the application of the right to life to suicide prevention is uncertain (*Rabone and another* (*Appellants*) *v Pennine Care NHS Trust* (*Respondent*) [2012], UKSC, n.1), and that operational duties will develop incrementally (*Daniel v. Saint George's Healthcare NHS Trust*, [2016], EWHC, 23 (QB)).

1.7   Good Samaritan Law

The question of when a person has a duty to act should be extended to the question of whether there is a duty to prevent or attempt to prevent a suicide. An intervention to prevent a suicide in the making or one that is anticipated brings to the surface unceasing and confrontational debates about the moral content of the law. In the twentieth century, the repeal in most countries of laws making it a criminal offence to attempt suicide (see Chapter 7) has led to a focus on the moral and legal obligations to rescue people who are on the verge of taking their own lives. Because suicide is a matter of life or death and there is something irksome about standing and watching it happen without intervention, the law in this instance is pushed to its limits with respect to 'justice' and 'mercy' as basic components of a legal system.

In the area of the duty to rescue, it has been a well-established perspective that European-oriented civil law has emanated from a communitarian approach and therefore is logically connected to an interventionist modality with penal consequences. In contrast, Anglo-Saxon common-law history has emphasised autonomy and freedom of action over and against social responsibility.

Common law, in contrast to civil law, does not have a universal criminal liability for the failure to act. As an example of a common-law country, in the United States (USA) there are civil statutes granting a form of immunity from civil liability when rescuing a person. In these statutes, professionals are sometimes subject to different and higher standards than volunteering individuals. One author has divided the variations into three categories: full liability protection, limited liability protection, and no liability protection (Northcut, 2018). Apart from such legislation, common-law judges have delineated specific rules: Once a person begins a rescue, it must not be discontinued, and the tort-feasor (person who commits a tort) is only held accountable for the injuries if the situation is worsened (Dawson, 1960). In common law there are additional special rules, such as those pertaining to property owners, parents, lifeguards, security officers, and lately there is an application of US law to the rescue of migrants (Post *et al.*, 2003).

Almost one-third of US states – California, Colorado, Florida, Massachusetts, Ohio, Minnesota, Nevada, Alaska, Hawaii, Rhode Island, Texas, Vermont, Washington, and Wisconsin – have criminalised failure to act, and each state has a different approach to penalties and criteria. The statutory varieties, both for civil immunity and penal responsibility, create some uncertainty in the USA, as the location is paramount for understanding the prospect of liability. A number of states have specified that individuals are required to assist when they are aware that another person is in danger, and that they may assist without creating danger to themselves or others.

Historically, in the civil law countries criminal statutes were first enacted under autocratic or dictatorial regimes. They used duty-to-rescue laws as a vehicle to encourage citizens to inform on each other, as in Vichy France under the domination of the Nazis or the infamous periods of the former Soviet Union. In this case the statutes were a lure for individuals to denounce those disloyal to the existing powers (Hayden, 2000). Following these ironic beginnings, by the end of the twentieth century laws about a duty to rescue were encapsulated into the majority of European juris-dictions. Despite this, punitive sanctions have generally been light, and there are no differential patterns in their application worthy of our atten-tion (Feinberg, 1980; Feldbrugge, 1965). The current situation is as follows: Whether in civil or common-law jurisdictions, the courts have not used serious criminal sanctions in the application of statutes and codes unless circumstances were seen as heinous in the public eye.

An additional factor related to holding someone responsible for failure to act is the broadly accepted psychological understanding that bystanders are wont to panic, making it difficult to isolate blameworthiness within a crowd. Only in a small minority of cases do we find an outcome of paying damages, and that has happened where interventions have indeed done more harm than good, causing substantial losses. In sum, spontaneous al-truism is honoured as an act of charity or as a moral duty from a variety of perspectives. Regardless of whether this positive appreciation stems from deontological libertarian, or relativist/contextual (utilitarian) standpoints, it is difficult to identify likely naysayers regarding the attractive quality of intervening to save the lives of strangers. We can turn to mass media to be confirmed in this generalisation.

How does this lend itself to our valuing voluntary, nonpaying acts, as dis-tinct from assistance rendered by professionals, who are compensated for their services? Some commentators have used arguments, even Kantian ones, to oppose a duty to rescue in tort law because of the commitment that the voluntariness should rest in the private sphere and never be made a legal duty (Uelmen, 2016; Volokh, 1999).

Tort law in common-law countries has consistently differentiated between those who have had professional training and laypeople, requiring the former to be held to a higher professional standard. For people with pro-fessional training, if there is a failure to perform the function according to the reasonable standard of those similarly trained, then liability results. To date, there is no body of material to which we can refer when making dis-tinctions between professionals and laypeople in determining liabilities for suicide rescuers.

In the practice of suicide prevention helplines, the distinction between the roles of professionals and laypeople is often blurred, with each having identical responsibility to help and save the lives of suicidal persons. Crisis and suicide prevention helplines worldwide are divided among centres that pay professional counsellors and centres that rely upon trained lay volunteers to answer calls and respond to chat and text messages from suicidal individuals. Since lives are at stake regardless of the professional status of helpers, are we to conclude that liability should be equal? This argument is bolstered by research findings over fifty years that show that lay volunteers are superior to more highly trained professionals such as psychiatrists, psychologists, and social workers when it comes to helping suicidal people through helplines.

A seminal article by Durlak (1979) reviewed 42 studies comparing the effectiveness of professional and nonprofessional helpers with respect to outcomes. The research found that nonprofessionals had equal or better clinical outcomes than the professionals. Later, Hattie and Hansford (1984) conducted meta-analyses of 154 comparisons in 39 studies and concluded that nonprofessionals were more likely to achieve resolution of the person's problems than professionals were. Mishara *et al.* (2016) found that more recent studies underscored that help provided by lay volunteers was at least as effective, and in most cases more effective, than the responses of professionals. These research studies used a variety of indicators of the effectiveness of interventions, ranging from client survey reports on the perceived helpfulness of the session, to decreases in suicide risk, and behaviours measured with standardised scales and observations. No matter which criteria were used, the lay volunteers were found to be as effective as professionals, and usually better. These research findings suggest that there is no evidence of different abilities in preventing suicides between trained laypeople and professionals that would justify having different levels of responsibility for these two groups.

It is important to recognise that the prediction of who is at high risk of suicidal behaviour lacks specificity and sensitivity. Even when using the best diagnostic tools currently available, there is always a large number of false positives (people being identified as about to attempt suicide who do not initiate an attempt) and false negatives (people who are thought to be at low risk who proceed with a suicide attempt). (See Chapter 2 for a detailed discussion of this.)

In the common-law area, a landmark article, 'The Case for a Duty to Rescue' by E. J. Weinrib, appeared in the *Yale Law Journal* in 1980, which looked into the growth of case law to tease out a 'rule of obligation' to intervene when there would be limited loss or difficulty. This work morally highlighted the case of the 'easy rescue'. In the words of Professor Weinrib:

> When there is an emergency that the rescuer can alleviate with no inconvenience to himself, the general duty of beneficence that is suspended over society like a floating charge is temporarily revealed to identify a particular obligor and obligee, and to define obligations that are specific enough for judicial enforcement. ... That tort law's adoption of a duty of easy rescue in emergencies would fit a common-law pattern ... that gives expression to the law's understanding of liberty. (Weinrib, 1980, p. 293)

Since the 1980s, there has not been an articulated rule accepted as the 'common rule of the common law'.

The role of tort principles is important in understanding how the law of Good Samaritanship has evolved in parallel with civil and penal statutes. Common law has increasingly focused on autonomy and freedom, as opposed to collective morality, as the prevailing reference point (Linden, 1972; Montana, 2017). In the final analysis, common sense is the best predictor of how emerging cases will be decided upon, regardless of the jurisdiction, civil or common law. One component is whether to define duty to rescue from a theory of contract law as opposed to tort law (Eisenberg, 2002; Scordato, 2008).

In tort law there is a necessity of locating a duty, wherever possible a reasonable standard of care, a proof of causation, and the link between the actor and the result in terms of any harm (damages) being inflicted. Where there is no cause, there is no tort. Normally, the language deployed is one of proximate causation, with this test linked to the language of foreseeability and risk. Without specific legislation demanding that morality be incorporated into civil law or common-law traditions, despite the many efforts of legal academics and philosophers of law, the status quo has essentially remained.

In our contemporary global period of anonymity in the digital universe, exacerbated by the COVID-19 pandemic, is it time for the courts and the legislatures to move forward towards some unanimity in encouraging suicide prevention? Should we advance our thinking internationally to forgive even acts of negligence where the intent was to do good rather than to induce or create harm? Should governments guarantee that professional groups doing suicide prevention be properly insured? Should lay volunteers, who constitute a large proportion of the counsellors in suicide prevention helplines and providers of online interventions to prevent suicides, have special protections to compensate for their lack of insurance and support from a professional association or licensing body? Our position is that such movements should be encouraged through effective lobbying and international cooperation.

We contend that legal considerations rarely resolve ethical dilemmas; when meaningful resolution occurs, it is usually determined by internalised ethical standards. We now turn to an examination of some of those issues and dilemmas.

2

• • • • • • •

Moral Dilemmas in Helpline Rescue Policies

As we have seen in Chapter 1, philosophical arguments concerning the morality of suicide have been one of the major themes in ethical philosophy throughout history. Yet few of the philosophers who argued eloquently about whether suicide is morally acceptable have themselves been faced with practical decisions concerning what to do when confronted with a suicidal individual. In this chapter we examine a range of contemporary ethical dilemmas faced by individuals working in suicide prevention, using crisis or suicide helplines as a case study. We analyse and contrast the ethical foundations in the policies of the Samaritans in the United Kingdom (UK) and those of the National Suicide Prevention Lifeline (NSPL, 988) helplines network in the United States (USA), expanding upon Mishara and Weisstub (2010). We focus on policies concerning the circumstances under which the emergency rescue of a caller to a telephone, chat, or text-message helpline is undertaken, if such emergency rescues are undertaken at all. Through the lenses of moralism, relativism, and libertarianism (see Chapter 1), we see that implicit and explicit ethical premises can be used to justify differing emergency rescue policies. Practical arguments based on empirically assessable impacts play a lesser but nonetheless important role in justifying policies and practices.

2.1   Positions of Telephone Helpline Organisations

Organisations offering suicide prevention services differ in the extent of their perceived obligations to intervene. These differences are based on fundamental beliefs concerning the limits of the respect of the free will to end one's life and the possible obligation to save a life, even against a person's wishes.

One example is the position concerning interventions with suicidal people held by the Samaritans organisation (Samaritans, 2020). Suicide prevention centres following the Samaritans model were originally developed in England by the late Anglican minister Chad Varah. England and the Republic of Ireland presently have over 200 branches of the Samaritans, with over 30,000 volunteers. Organisations that are affiliated with Befrienders Worldwide follow broad Samaritans principles but may differ in some practices; they include 349 member centres in 32 different countries, which offer telephone help for suicidal people, face-to-face meetings, as well as email and rapidly expanding short message service (SMS) text messages and chat services. The basic mission of the Samaritans is to alleviate emotional distress and reduce the incidence of suicidal feelings and suicidal behaviour (Samaritans, 2020). The Samaritans' vision is to promote societies in which fewer people die by suicide. Despite this primary objective, they uphold the premise that everyone has the right to make fundamental decisions about their own lives, including the decision to die by suicide.

These principles have been interpreted to imply that extraordinary means, such as sending an ambulance when a person's life is at risk from a suicide attempt, may not be undertaken *unless it is the client's decision to get help*. Although some Samaritans centres engage in rescue activities when an explicit request for help is not received, other centres cite this principle to justify their non-intervention with people who say that they have decided to end their own lives. Some centres report 'accompanying' an adult who has initiated a suicide attempt and does not want the attempt stopped, by simply talking with the caller while the person is in the process of dying.

Although this may appear to be a callous approach in which suicidal people are just 'left to die', in reality it is the experience of Samaritans organisations that most people, once they begin to talk about their distress and despair, become less suicidal, and that those who are still at high risk or have initiated an attempt generally ask for or accept help that is offered. The Samaritans see the process of respecting the caller's wishes as having the positive effect in their suicide prevention activities of providing non-judgemental support. They believe that people have the right to find their own solution and that telling people what to do takes responsibility and moral agency away from them. It is rare that callers do not change their minds about killing themselves in the process of discussions with Samaritans volunteers. However, the principle that the decision to die by suicide must be respected remains a primary reference within the organisation. Even so, the UK Samaritans have been considering future directions in which the obligation to respect the decision to die by suicide is not practiced.

The Samaritans justify their policy of respecting the suicidal intentions of callers and not intervening against the wishes of a caller in two ways. First, they adopt an explicit libertarian ethical stance in which they believe that the decision to live or die rests with the caller and that telephone helpers should not contravene an individual's decision under any circumstances. However, it is not clear whether this respect for the caller's decision to live or die is superseded when there is blatant evidence of incoherence, mental illness, or intoxication discernible during the call.

Second, the Samaritans use a consequentialist argument to justify their respect for the caller's wishes. They say that people in distress call the Samaritans with the knowledge that the content of their conversations is confidential and that they will be able to maintain total anonymity. They contend that if confidentiality were to be broken in some instances to rescue a caller who has decided to attempt suicide, this violation of their 'contract' could discourage other callers from contacting them and receiving help when they are in need.

2.2   The American Association of Suicidology and the US National Suicide Prevention Lifeline Network Positions

The American Association of Suicidology (AAS), which certifies many suicide prevention and crisis centres in the USA, and the National Suicide Prevention Lifeline (NSPL) network, which coordinates centres across the USA linked to the central toll-free number 988, have policies that contrast with the Samaritans' respect for the decision to die by suicide. The certified centres are evaluated by on-site visits, where they are expected to meet stringent standards concerning their policies, procedures, and methods of intervention. Among the obligations of AAS accreditation and NSPL policies is the necessity to provide 'rescue services' and to intervene in life-threatening crises along with other community resources such as health and safety agencies. Centres must have a well-planned rescue capacity, which is documented in writing and adhered to consistently. According to the guidelines, centres must 'at the very least, be capable of initiating or actually accomplishing a rescue intervention in cases of life-threatening acts already set into motion' (American Association of Suicidology, 2017, p. 58). Rescue is a response to a cry for help and may often involve taking extraordinary actions to save a life. Rescue procedures typically involve tracing calls, informing police and ambulance services, sending a mental health crisis team to the person's location, and entering a person's home to prevent their death by suicide, with or without the person's permission.

The NSPL has developed 'Policies and Standards for Helping Callers at Imminent Risk of Suicide', which require members of the network to take the most collaborative and least invasive course of action to protect the health, safety, and well-being of the callers to their helplines (Draper *et al.*, 2015). Although they do everything possible to obtain the at-risk individual's cooperation, member centres are obliged to facilitate 'active rescue' life-saving services on the client's behalf if their client is attempting suicide or are at 'imminent risk' of suicide, even when the caller refuses to have help sent. This obligation includes having access to Caller ID, tracing calls, geo-localisation of portable cell phones, Internet use locations, having supervisory staff available for consultation at all times, contacting emergency medical services with whom they have an agreement so that these services can intervene with the caller, confirming emergency services contacts, and active follow-up when emergency services are unsuccessful.

It is the experience of the centres that these procedures are rarely used. In most circumstances where callers initially refuse medical help or other interventions to prevent their death, after they talk with a telephone worker the callers eventually change their mind and ask for rescue services or accept that help be sent.

Although there is no specific statement of ethical, philosophical, or moral belief that justifies the position of the AAS or the NSPL, there is an implicit moralist stance. They assume that if a life is in danger, a rescue must be undertaken in all circumstances, even where the caller explicitly states that they do not want to be rescued. Some NSPL centres also justify their rescue procedures by a consequentialist argument that is different from that of the Samaritans' philosophy. AAS centres report that callers who are rescued against their will often phone back later to thank the centre for saving their lives. They contend that since many people are pleased that they were rescued, this indicates that the people were 'not themselves' or in a clear state of mind when they initiated their suicide attempts. In effect, the Samaritans and the NSPL centres use competing anecdotal evidence to support contrasting moral approaches to intervention.

2.3   Legal Imperatives, Jurisprudence, and Leeway Given to Helpers

Several organisations skirt the moral issue of whether one should rescue a caller during an attempt by insisting that what they are doing is following the legal prescripts of their country or state. However, as pointed out previously (see Chapter 1), Good Samaritan Laws that obligate citizens to assist or locate help for people whose lives are in danger are almost never invoked to obligate actions. They have served mainly to protect people who intervene to save a life from prosecution or civil damages.

Even when there are clear institutional policies mandating emergency rescues during a suicide attempt, individual helpline workers often express a contextualist approach in which they believe there are situations when the decision to end one's life should be respected and emergency rescue should not be sent. Usually these instances concern elderly and/or terminally ill people who are suffering. The extent to which the feelings expressed by helpline workers influence whether emergency rescue is actually sent is not yet known. Whenever he presents a workshop or conducts training of telephone helpline workers, one of the authors (BLM) invariably encounters people who adhere to the relativist–contextualist position of being less inclined to want to rescue when the person is elderly, severely disabled, or terminally ill.

2.4   Imminent But Not Immediate Acts

Situations become more complex when the caller is not in the process of an act that is life-threatening, but an attempt appears to be imminent. The USA's NSPL policy stipulates that people who are assessed to be at imminent risk of attempting suicide should be sent emergency rescue, even against the caller's expressed wishes, if the helper is convinced that the person's life will probably be in danger in the near future. The NSPL defines imminent risk as existing when the Centre Staff responding to the call believes there is a close temporal connection between the person's current risk status and actions that could lead to his/her suicide, or believes that if no action were taken, the caller would be likely to seriously harm or kill him/her self. The NSPL further stipulates that imminent risk may be determined if an individual states (or is reported to have stated by a person believed to be a reliable informant) both a desire and an intent to die and has the capability of carrying out his or her intent (Draper *et al.*, 2015).

In order to understand the ethical issues concerning rescue against a caller's wish when an attempt appears to be imminent but is not in process, we need to consider several issues. The first is to question the extent to which one can reliably know that a caller will attempt suicide when the attempt has not yet been initiated. Suicidology research on prediction indicates that we are not yet able to provide even near certitude in determining if or when a person will attempt suicide. This then raises the issue of the validity of risk assessments: To what extent are telephone helpers' evaluations of the probability of an imminent attempt accurate? To date, we have no empirical evidence to justify that telephone helpers are capable of predicting which callers will or will not attempt suicide.

In any situation where one wishes to predict behaviour on the basis of present experiences or information obtained at a given point in time, uncertainty remains. Human beings do not always do what we think they will do, although we may have the most accurate prediction tools available. This is both because the prediction tools have a large margin of error, and because people may act irrationally or change their plans without notice. Even the person who is fixated on suicide, has written a suicide note, and has prepared a plan may very well change their course of action in midstream. Equally, a person who is evaluated as having a low suicide risk could subsequently experience a dramatic negative change in circumstances and, if there is ready access to a means of suicide, could initiate a lethal suicide attempt without notice.

One may also ask what effect sending some form of emergency rescue will have on the lives of callers, both those who are truly planning an imminent suicide, and those who are not truly in physical danger but have been erroneously identified as being at high risk. People who are sent to an emergency room, based on the conviction of a helper that they are going to attempt suicide later, may simply convince the emergency help that there is nothing wrong. If they are brought to a hospital, they may simply be returned home immediately if there are no signs of wounds and if the person has denied suicidal intentions. Thus, the emergency rescue, which hoped to interrupt a dangerous process, may not have any positive effect on the person's suicidal plans. Those who are sent to hospital without having initiated an attempt are still in a vulnerable situation. One could even wonder if their suicidal intentions are strengthened by the experience of their autonomy being violated, or by the subsequent stigma of having the experience exposed to friends and relatives. Empirical evidence would be of use to guide us in addressing these dilemmas. However, data on the effects of emergency interventions are sorely lacking. Currently, emergency interventions are undertaken based on the implicit assumptions that the emergency rescue will be helpful, and that those instances when emergency rescue is sent inappropriately do not create significant undue harm. These are assumptions that should be clarified by research.

2.5   Salient Questions

Analogous to what occurs in the field of applied bioethics, the challenge for actors in the field of suicide prevention is how to meaningfully link assertions about principles or fundamental values to particular actions. The move from the abstract to the real is often fraught with contradictory nuances and conflicts about competing values stemming from personal background, religious upbringing, identification with the interests of a cultural minority, or personal experiences of a traumatic nature.

In fact, there are two sets of issues about how fundamental values come into play. First, there is the commitment that an organisational entity such as the Samaritans, the American Association of Suicidology, or the US National Suicide Prevention Lifeline has made in their statements of purpose and how their administrators implement these moral principles and fundamental values, which have a multiplicity of origins. Second, there is the matter of the cultural factors in specific legal and political contexts that can bear down heavily on the perspective of both nationally based organisations and individual citizens.

One question is whether it is possible to make generalisations about the governing values of the organisations based on their rescue policies. Perhaps the more pressing question is whether the apparent differences of orientation with respect to rescue policies as expressed by the Samaritans, the American Association of Suicidology, and the US NSPL may be more theoretical than real.

We could assert that the American-based position seems to be moralistically driven, because their intervention style is more aggressive than the Samaritans' counterpart. The American organisations' more interventionist policies are based on the moral mandate to save a life whenever possible, even if it requires violations of privacy or autonomy. The collective responsibility to protect the sanctity of life is seen as deriving from natural law, which for some has a higher ontological status than any given mores of a culture or constitutional legal values expressed at any given moment. It may be equally plausible that the interventionist American model is driven by a strong collectivist instinct in the culture of self-preservation. Admittedly, the notion of the collective good may be fuelled more by its defensive utilitarianism than by any kind of universalist Kantian standard (see Chapter 1), or even a sense of Christian values. Having said that, it is not difficult to see that human rights advocates find themselves at loggerheads with comparable activists on the other side of a constitutional pendulum, who are prepared to go to great ends in order to preserve life.

Similarly, we are hard-pressed to know precisely how to generalise about the Samaritans' work under the rubric of their founding mandate, either in legal–cultural terms or in reference to the social values that are deployed by the actors in the system. The difference between the two models addressed in this chapter may, in the final analysis, be one of degree rather than one of kind. It is plausible that an overwhelming number of people working in suicide prevention harbour commitments, indeed akin to the organisations that they represent, that walk a difficult line between moralistic impulses and pragmatic requirements. The connectors between the two suggest that most practitioners can be legitimately described as contexualists; what pretty much everyone shares in rescuing lives is the view that suicide is almost always an act that goes against the best interests of the individual and the social network that surrounds the person.

The Samaritans may contend that the long-term viability of the organisation depends on maintaining a credible respect for the decisions of callers. In the US centres, they may feel that it is essential to engage in active rescues to preserve their perceived role for the general public and to sustain their credibility with politically motivated funders. Regardless of the policy approach used, people who actively participate in suicide prevention share the desire to save lives. We must be cautious in asserting that differences in rescue policies reflect fundamental differences in orientation or in commitment to the goal of providing help.

Is it possible to ask leading international organisations to better clarify their first principles? Or should we conclude that such a venture would be misguided because we need to acknowledge that people working in the field of suicide prevention are forced by the very nature of their craft to inhabit a middle territory where principles and pragmatism coalesce? Active debate is needed on this subject in order to unpack how essential or real the divergences are. The research on these questions is inadequate. We know little about how the current actors in the field appreciate the nature of ethical challenges and the contradictions that arise.

Finally, we know that the relationship between suicide and mental disorder is significant. Nevertheless, we are obligated to probe the parameters of autonomy when rationality is claimed. Because of this fact, societies, whether countries living in the Anglo-Saxon legal tradition or in that of Continental Europe, will find extreme permissiveness an anathema to their prevailing moral sensibilities. The dominant international organisations in suicide prevention continue to share the presumption that saving lives from suicide is a worthwhile and justifiable social endeavour. Their pursuits should not be held back, even if one believes that there is compelling evidence that autonomy must be respected in a small minority of cases where it may be possible to justify taking of one's life, either through cool philosophical reflection or because of extraordinary conditions that have made life unbearable. For the rest, there will be ongoing debates about the best strategies for effective intervention.

We conclude that it is necessary that a vigorous dialogue about values be sustained in order that all parties to the debate – organisations and individuals included – be sensitised to the role that values play in applying institutional philosophies in the face of hard cases in the grey zones of moral practice.

3

• • • • • • •

Ethical Challenges
in Suicide Research

3.1 Vulnerability

Suicide is related to vulnerability in the sense that people struggling with suicidality fall into the classification of vulnerability as understood by such bodies as the Council for International Organizations of Medical Sciences, which in collaboration with the World Health Organization have issued 'International Ethical Guidelines for Biomedical Research Involving Human Subjects' (Council for International Organizations of Medical Sciences (CIOMS), 2016, p. 110). In the view of this body, vulnerability is associated with substantial incapacity to protect one's own interests, which can relate to a wide variety of problems. Such vulnerability can happen to an individual, as in nontherapeutic experimentation, where vulnerability is the inability to protect oneself from exposure to an unreasonable risk of harm. At a group level, vulnerability can occur when a minority group is treated unequally based on group membership. For vulnerable groups who face systematic discrimination, questions arise concerning voluntariness and the capacity to provide valid and informed consent to participate in research. In the case of potentially suicidal individuals, who are by definition vulnerable, we can never be certain whether our interventions are intrinsically paternalistic and thereby morally unacceptable, or whether the person in crisis can give meaningful consent to participate. Our social instinct is to regard the vast majority of suicidal individuals as vulnerable but also to seek to intervene.

A common focus of suicide-related research is to study the extent of people's vulnerability, expressed as suicide risk. Suicidal populations often overlap with other vulnerable groups – such as those with mental illness, people who have experienced traumatic events, and the elderly – who present specific challenges. The moral arguments that arise in research with such populations are further complicated in suicide research (Fitzpatrick, 2021; Weisstub, 2001; Weisstub and Thomasma, 2001).

Research in suicide is often difficult to separate from therapeutic interests. Conducting pure research in suicidology may be an ideal that is impossible to achieve. Obviously, no suicidal participants should ever be placed in a no-treatment control group in a randomised trial. It would be considered inhumane to study individuals with life-threatening suffering without helping or offering help. The justification of research becomes a serious challenge when nontherapeutic research on potentially vulnerable populations is conducted.

In the name of the principle of justice, the Belmont Report in 1978 required that subjects be selected for 'reasons directly related to the problem being studied' rather than 'simply because of their easy availability, their compromised position, or their manipulability' (National Commission for the Protection of Human Subjects of Biomedical and Behavioral Research, 1979, p. 10). In the discussion of suicidology research that follows, vulnerability is a recurrent theme that is often the principal cause of concern, particularly vulnerability from having an increased risk of suicide.

3.2   Experimental Methodologies

For many, the gold standard for research on efficacy of a treatment is to conduct a random assignment study in which participants who are assigned to an experimental condition receive a treatment and those assigned to a control condition receive either no treatment or a placebo condition that has no known specific effect related to the outcomes under investigation. In the case of suicide research, experimental methodologies involving no-treatment control groups are rarely used because of ethical concerns. It is generally considered unethical to assign a no-treatment control condition to individuals who may be at risk of suicide in order to determine if an experimental treatment has a preventive effect for others. Because of this concern, it is common practice to exclude potentially suicidal individuals from participating in studies evaluating the effectiveness of new medications. This has resulted in the curious phenomenon that new drugs developed to treat mental health problems, which are commonly used in the treatment of suicidal individuals, are not initially tested with people at risk of suicide. The suicide of a study participant may or may not be related to the intervention, making it more difficult to assess the effect of the intervention. There are also legal concerns. If people die by suicide in the course of research evaluating a new medication, the drug company may be held liable for their deaths.

An alternative to using a no-treatment control condition is to compare a new treatment with 'treatment as usual', TAU (Degenholtz *et al.*, 2002; Fisher *et al.*, 2002; Saigle *et al.*, 2017). If there is no reason to assume on the basis of existing knowledge ('theoretical equipoise') that the new treatment is better, and there is a debate among clinicians as to which treatment is best ('clinical equipoise', Freedman, 1987), one may assume that TAU methodologies do not expose the control group to added risks (Andriessen *et al.*, 2019). However, in a situation where differences between treatments are not known, there is a potential risk in participating in any new treatment in the experimental group, and there is a potential risk of being deprived of a beneficial intervention in the control group. After all, the researchers would not be undertaking the investigation if they did not have good reason to believe that the new treatment given to the experimental group offers significant benefits.

From a strict moralist point of view, exclusion of people from experimental methodologies that employ no-treatment or placebo controls is seen as essential, because the obligation to protect people from suicide and preserve life is the highest priority. Where there is a risk of suicide, intervention is required. TAU studies, in which all participants receive some 'treatment as usual' may be acceptable. However, recent studies suggest that some standard treatments, for instance the use of the new generation of medications such as venlafaxine for the treatment of depression, may not be effective in decreasing suicide risk and may even increase suicides in adolescents (Hengartner *et al.*, 2021; Hetrick *et al.*, 2021). In this instance moralists would insist that only known effective or recommended treatments be always made available.

From a libertarian perspective, the right of individuals to choose to live or die includes the right to choose whether to put health and life at potential risk by participating in a research study involving a no-treatment control group. Moralists could approve of such a randomised control research design if the choice to risk no-treatment was consciously made in order to potentially advance knowledge and benefit humanity by preserving the lives of others in the future.

Contextualists in the relativist camp, who believe that the circumstances can determine what is ethically correct (see Chapter 1), would assess the ethics of experimental methods in each particular instance. For example, one can weigh the potential risks to participants in an experimental investigation against the potential benefits for those who could eventually benefit from the research results. This type of analysis can only take place when there are sufficient data available to determine potential risks and benefits.

In the case of testing established treatments in TAU designs where some data are available, there may be a basis for undertaking an analysis of the possible risks and advantages. However, in the case of new interventions not previously evaluated, any analysis would have to be based on hypothetical beliefs or clinical judgements about what should or should not be helpful in specific situations. Furthermore, the practical issue of how to balance the potential benefits of potential future lives saved against possible risks of lives lost to suicide remains a controversial terrain on which no guidelines currently exist. Still, it is possible that the risks, which would be of concern for relativist/contextualists and moralists, may be decreased by the inclusion of increased surveillance of participants in a research study and the inclusion of rescue procedures.

3.3   Rescue Procedures

Most studies on suicide include some criteria for rescue of a potentially suicidal person (Andriessen *et al.*, 2019; Packman and Harris, 1998). Participants in studies, without explicitly seeking intervention or prevention, may divulge information that indicates that they or a third party is a suicide risk. This would require that researchers refer to an intervention procedure should a life be deemed endangered in the course of the study.

Neither researchers nor clinicians are currently able to accurately identify all people at significant risk of self-injury or suicide (Chandler *et al.*, 2021; Hawton *et al.*, 1998; Kessler *et al.*, 2020). One of the important challenges in developing any rescue criteria is to determine to what extent false positives and false negatives are acceptable. It could be argued that implementation of more-inclusive rescue or intervention standards might deflect energies to low-risk individuals while at the same time missing some people who are truly suicidal.

Moralists would contend that it is imperative to include intervention and rescue criteria that are as sensitive as possible, in order to identify and save as many lives as possible. The dangers of subjecting some people who are not actually at risk to intrusive interventions are seen by moralists as minimal in comparison with the potential to save a life.

Libertarians would not ever instigate rescue or intervention procedures against the will of the participant. However, libertarians could respect existing guidelines by including a protocol where anyone found to be at risk would be informed about potential sources of help and, if the participant so chose, the researchers could assist them in obtaining help. Even the staunchest libertarian would probably agree that information about potential sources of help should be given, with the participant in the research being free to contact or not the source of help if the person so chose.

The relativist could weigh the pros and cons, risks and benefits of various rescue procedures, given the risks of false positives and false negatives. Nevertheless, the relativist's analysis would be limited by the lack of specific knowledge of the risks and benefits, due to the unreliability of suicide risk assessment procedures and our inability to accurately predict treatment outcomes.

One of the practical challenges to including rescue and intervention procedures in research protocols relates to the clinical skills of the researchers. Some suicidology researchers are skilled clinicians with good diagnostic and intervention skills. Other suicidology researchers do not have this background and would not be capable of intervening or conducting a good clinical assessment. In these instances, there may be an obligation for researchers without clinical expertise to have clinicians or suicide prevention organisations involved, or at least available, to intervene in suicidal crisis situations that may occur in the course of the study.

3.4   Obtaining Informed Consent

One of the basic requirements in conducting ethical research is the obligation to obtain the informed consent of participants in which confidentiality is guaranteed. Confidentiality is also an explicit part of the mutual agreement between clients and helpers in many suicide prevention settings. In studies of high-risk vulnerable individuals, however, complete confidentiality is usually not guaranteed. Typically, there are policies that determine the conditions for breaking the confidentiality agreement in order to initiate rescues to save a life (see Chapter 2 for discussion of helpline rescue procedures). For example, calls to a suicide crisis line involve an interaction with a helper, in which confidence is developed and intimate details of the caller's life are revealed.

Obtaining informed consent for research purposes may compromise the intervention process. Imagine beginning a call from a person in a suicidal crisis line with: 'Before we begin to discuss your problems, I would like to invite you to participate in a research study where people will be listening to the calls and assessing various characteristics of the helper and caller. This study is being conducted by Researcher X and has the objective of determining the effectiveness of the help provided ...' Following such an introduction, lengthy information about confidentiality, whom to contact if there are issues about the research, etc., the objectives of the study, and the possible risks and benefits would be disclosed. Only after the aforementioned transaction would the conversation give help to the suicidal caller.

The many details and the length of time involved in obtaining the caller's consent to participate in the study could have a negative impact on the callers' abilities to access immediate help for their problems in a secure and supportive context. The helpers, who are fully aware that someone is listening to the call, may be overly tense or anxious about the researcher's assessment, thus hampering the helpers' ability to interact in the most helpful manner. Moreover, if such procedures were instituted, the result would be a likely sampling bias in which only those callers who are not in an urgent crisis would agree to participate. Informed consent may also be compromised by the desperate need of some callers to obtain help and the fear that the helper or the response to their plight will be influenced by whether they choose to participate in the research.

A strongly moralist position would suggest that anything that might impinge on the ability of suicidal people to obtain help should not be undertaken. This imperative may be challenged by the potentially life-saving value of obtaining nonbiased evaluations of the quality of help received by suicidal people. Sacrificing the obligation for informed consent by listening to calls without informing callers or helpers might offer better-quality services. However, current ethical guidelines usually mandate obtaining consent from all research participants. A compromise position might be to have a recorded announcement informing callers that their call 'may be monitored', so at least callers would be made aware of the potential of third-party monitoring.

A libertarian could approach this situation from various perspectives. The libertarian might feel it is essential that a suicidal person have the free choice to participate – or not participate – in any research study, and that full explanations and informed consent are essential. However, a libertarian could equally hold that people experiencing a suicidal crisis should have the liberty to seek help to resolve their crises without the interference of intrusive research practises. Libertarians might therefore not accept any practises that compromise the quality of the help that callers should be able to receive. Like some moralists, libertarians could be concerned that if research were not conducted, this would block the improvement of services to people who contact a helpline in the future.

Relativists would inevitably weigh the potential benefits against the potential harm caused by various practises. They might compare the possible dangers of conducting a research investigation in which data are obtained on someone without their consent to the potential benefits of doing so, or might look at the relative harm of providing information to obtain informed consent versus the potential benefits of the study, etc. Alas, it is often the case that there are insufficient data to support such analyses. In a silent monitoring study (Mishara *et al.*, 2007), the decision was made to inform callers in a recorded announcement of the possibility that calls were monitored preceding their connection to the helper at the crisis line. In initial discussions of this practice with crisis centres, many helpers were concerned that callers who heard this announcement would hang up and would not receive critical assistance. It should be noted, however, that crisis centres that already used such recorded messages reported no increase in hang-ups, except possibly a decrease in the number of 'sex' calls. Empirical assessments during the course of the study did not indicate any increase in hang-ups when this message was included. In this instance, admittedly, there were data available from previous studies. However, there are many areas for which no previous experience exists. In these cases, one may argue about potential consequences, but the basis for decisions remains speculative.

3.5   Deception and Disclosure

Studies involving deceptive practices have generally been justified as causing minimal or no harm, being necessary when no other means of obtaining the information without deception is available, and needed when the information sought is judged to be of high scientific or practical value. In the case of the silent monitoring of calls to crisis centres, one of the methodological procedures proposed to assess the quality of services while avoiding the problems involved in informed consent procedures was to have a trained actor place fictional calls to crisis centres. It was proposed that a skilled actor pretend to be a suicidal person in crisis, and researchers would monitor those calls. If the goal is to evaluate the quality of telephone interventions – if helpers do what they are supposed to be doing to help suicidal callers according to generally accepted models of intervention and they have beneficial characteristics, such as empathy – this method of having 'false' calls might obtain this information in a relatively simple manner. This procedure was proposed to be used only if the actor were convincing and the helpers who received the calls did not know that these were not 'real' calls.

Although no suicidal person is directly in danger when fictitious calls are used, some risks may be identified. First, this practice involves deception of helpers. Also, during a fictional call real suicidal people might not have access to the helper who is occupied with the fictional caller. This could put suicidal individuals at greater risk if it compromises their ability to receive immediate help in a crisis situation. Furthermore, helpers should have the right to freely consent to participate in a research project. If they were informed that the caller was an actor, their intervention might be different. Finally, these calls are not without potential negative consequences. Helpers may experience the added stress of having to handle additional calls from people they think are really at risk, imminent or otherwise.

Moralists may justify such deception and lack of informed consent by citing their primary concern for saving lives. However, if there is a possibility that lives may be lost because the helper is occupied with a fictitious call, moralists may not be in favour of this practice. In their analysis, they might find themselves weighing the potential risks against the potential benefits in order to make a decision, and thus find themselves sliding towards a more relativist stance. The libertarian would seem to want the helper to make a clear, informed choice as to whether to participate in the study or not. The relativists might find it hard to have sufficient data to evaluate the advantages and disadvantages or consequences of this practice. It would be difficult to determine if the helpers were significantly stressed by the calls without actually conducting the study and measuring their stress. In fact, we know very little about effects of stress on helpline workers. We also do not know with any certainty how important it is for a caller in a crisis to reach a helper immediately. Some people may feel that if help is not immediately available, the caller could be at risk of suicide. Others may view the suicidal crisis differently and may feel that those who would truly benefit from help are known to persistently call until help is obtained.

3.6   Innovative and Unproven Interventions

One of the greatest challenges in suicidology research is to test innovative and unproven interventions whose effects are yet unknown. Because of possible paradoxical effects of increasing suicide risk, there may be hesitation to try anything new or to conduct research on innovative practices. Although logical and theoretical justifications for practices may seem strong, there are known paradoxical effects in suicidology. For example, one may think that showing photographs of people who died by suicide in newspapers and magazines could dissuade potential victims because of the graphic depiction of death. However, research has determined that when photographs showing how people kill themselves are published, there is an increased likelihood of copycat suicides (Pirkis *et al.*, 2017; Stack, 2005). In the past, there was much reluctance to ask direct questions to depressed and vulnerable clients about whether or not they were thinking of killing themselves, because of the belief that this might 'put ideas in people's minds'. It is now generally accepted that asking direct questions does not increase suicide risk. In fact, asking direct questions is considered as essential in assessing suicide risk.

If we do not have any firm data on the effects of a practice, and if our main concern is protecting human life, there may be a general tendency to avoid trying something new because of the potential risks. The moralist who holds that life should be protected at all costs may be conflicted between the potential risks of an untried practice versus the imperative to find better ways to save people's lives. Libertarians may feel that people should choose for themselves whether new practices are acceptable. However, they may justifiably realise that people would not have sufficient information with which to choose. Even the relativists may find that there is little concrete information with which to make any form of contextual or consequentialist analysis.

3.7   Choice of Participants

We have already discussed the elimination of participants who are at risk of suicide from studies involving experimental methodologies. The potential dangers to participants are not limited to situations where there are treatment and no-treatment groups. Any gathering of research information may have an effect on the suicidal risk of a participant. Questioning research participants may bring up memories of the circumstances surrounding suicidal intentions or attempts. Talking about their situation may have benefits for a participant or may result in increased risk. Again, the empirical data are lacking in most situations, so researchers must rely on clinical insights or careful monitoring as a study progresses. The libertarian would feel that if informed consent is obtained, people can simply choose to participate and assume the risks. Moralists, on the other hand, may put more emphasis on the researcher's obligation to ensure that participants are not placed at greater risk. Relativists may emphasise the need for participants and researchers to measure risks and weigh them against possible benefits.

3.8   Disclosure of Information Concerning Suicide Risk of Third Parties

In the course of research on suicide, researchers may learn that specific individuals, families, or contexts carry with them a high risk of suicide. We have already discussed rescue and intervention procedures when a participant in a study is identified as likely to engage in suicidal behaviours.

Sometimes, the information obtained does not directly concern the participant, but concerns others. This is common in survey and interview studies where participants are asked about their contacts with suicidal people. A case in point: during an interview study on suicide, an adult participant confides that a family member appears to be at high risk of attempting suicide. Since confidentiality has been promised, researchers might limit their actions to informing the participant about sources of help, inviting the participant to contact those sources, and encouraging the person at risk to contact them as well. Do these actions satisfy the researchers' ethical obligations? Does the researcher have any further obligation, or are they limited by their confidentiality agreement?

Moralists at first blush might vote in favour of intervention, to push researchers to contact the person at risk, maintaining that the principle of confidentiality has a lower priority than the overriding obligation to protect human life. On reflection, the information, although it may seem reliable, will be exposed in many contexts as hearsay, and it may be coloured by the subjective interpretation of the informer. The researcher does not have direct information concerning the person who is possibly at risk. Would the moralist feel strongly that one should send rescue services for a person never encountered? The libertarian would want to respect the rights of the suspected suicidal individual and consider that all interventions that happen without the person directly requesting help would impinge on the person's liberty to choose. However, what if the situation is more complex? What if the third party is said to appear greatly distressed and is asking for help? Would it significantly alter the context if the person suffers from a serious mental health problem, for example, schizophrenia, and is hearing voices telling him to kill himself?

Are there circumstances where the commitment to liberty is compromised by a serious mental health problem? It is in fact rare to find libertarians who hold to an absolutist position in view of overwhelming evidence of clear and present mental distortion. For the relativist, one may wonder which variables could show that intervention is indicated or not. In a culture where privacy is strictly respected, would intervention be less appropriate than in another community where there is a high level of community interaction? Would it matter why the person was intending to suicide? If the person is dying from cancer and is 90 years old, would this be more likely to suggest nonintervention, compared with the response to a young professional in good health?

Special policies for research with minors (people under age 18 or 16, depending on the locality) recognise the developmental vulnerabilities of this population. Specific concerns have been encoded in laws that mandate disclosure of any dangers to a minor's physical or mental health. Age differences have no influence on the moralist position favouring any action that contributes to saving human life. The challenge for the libertarian perspective is to establish when a person has the capacity to make decisions that must be respected. Relativists would turn to any data available to determine whether the effects of identifying someone as suicidal and letting this be known to the family or helpers produces more risk than nonintervention.

3.9   At-Risk and Vulnerable Populations

The issue of inclusion of at-risk participants in a study and obtaining their informed consent becomes even more complicated with special populations, including children and emancipated minors, patients in psychiatric hospitals, prisoners, and people bereaved by suicide. External pressures in institutional settings, such as special privileges for prisoners or psychiatric patients who participate in research, pressure from staff who are in a powerful position, and feelings of guilt in those bereaved by suicide, may significantly influence the decision to participate in a research study. In these instances, one may question whether informed consent can ever be freely given. Is it ethical to test a potentially dangerous new intervention on prisoners in order to benefit the rest of society? Are prisoners, from a libertarian perspective, truly free to choose to participate in a research study? Should their lives be protected at all costs like anyone else's, as moralists might contend? Is the moralist position clear in its direction, given that a moralist might devalue rights based on the notion of social paybacks built into the equation of punishment? How does one calculate the relative benefits and for whom?

Very often issues concerning special populations are overly determined by existing legal constraints. The question of whether a person is legally competent to consent to participate in research may diverge from whether the person meets the ethical or functional criteria needed for competent decision-making. For example, in the case of emancipated minors, they may have the legal right to participate as adults, but there are indications that their rights need special protection by inclusion of child specialists in designing and evaluating research protocols (Rubinstein, 2003; Sadzaglishvili *et al.*, 2021).

Where data are lacking or unreliable, ethical choices are daunting from any perspective. For the moralist, it may not be an easy task to determine which behaviours should trigger interventions to protect life when they identify people as potentially suicidal. Relativists may find it hard to determine what to weigh in situations where few data are available. Libertarians may emphasise the importance of a person having the right to information as a basis for free and informed choice.

Ethicists may also examine the impact of any form of tests and measures for identifying who is suicidal. What constitutes sufficient accuracy and reliability to avoid the harms of false positives and false negatives for individuals, families, and society? Should one weigh the values of informing people of their diagnosis or of informing individuals, their families, or potential caregivers of their potential for suicide?

3.10 Indigenous Participants in Research

Indigenous Peoples, found in over 90 countries, constitute 6% of the world's population. They have repeatedly been subjected to experimentation without any of the concerns and precautions of modern enlightened ethical research practices, even when research on non-Indigenous Peoples observed strict ethical norms. The awareness of past abuses has led to the development of specific ethical guidelines for research with Indigenous Peoples to empower native, First Nation, Inuit, and other Indigenous Peoples to actively participate in the decision of whether and how to participate in a research project. An example is the specific policies of 'Research Involving the First Nations, Inuit and Métis People of Canada' of the Tri-Council Policy Statement *Ethical Conduct for Research Involving Human Subjects* (Canadian Institutes of Health Research & Natural Sciences and Engineering Research Council of Canada & Social Sciences and Humanities Research Council, 2018), which applies to all research funded by federal and provincial agencies in Canada. This ethics framework is based on three core ethical values: respect for persons, concern for welfare, and justice.

Respect for persons generally concerns securing free, informed, ongoing consent from participants. In the Indigenous context, this includes consideration of the interconnection between humans and the natural world and obligations to pass on to future generations knowledge received from ancestors as well as the knowledge developed in the present generation.

The welfare of individual participants that has been the major concern in other research projects must be expanded to concur with Indigenous world views, which consider individual participants in the context of their physical, social, economic, and cultural environments and the well-being of their whole community, and with respect for collective community rights. Research should not only respect, but should also enhance Indigenous People's capacities to maintain their cultures, languages, and identities.

The Tri-Council Policy Statement identifies specific challenges to ensuring justice in research, particularly where there exists an imbalance of power between the researcher and participants. In indigenous research settings, social, cultural, and linguistic differences, as well as historical mistrust between outside researchers and the community, can lead to difficulties in communication, mutual collaboration, and acceptance.

The guidelines require that Indigenous partners contribute to determining the nature, goals, and methods of the investigation and participate in collection, analysis, and interpretation of data. These guidelines indicate who 'owns' the data; it may be jointly owned by outside researchers and the participants' representatives or may be owned by the community or people under study. Rather than conducting research 'on' Indigenous People, enlightened researchers collaborate and co-develop research *with* Indigenous communities and focus on adapting research questions and practices to the cultural specificities and the needs of the community.

In 2023, the Global Alliance for Chronic Diseases (GACD), which supports implementation science research in seventy countries on noncommunicable diseases, including suicide, issued a statement on noncommunicable disease research with Indigenous Peoples (Meharg *et al.*, 2023). The statement, drafted by a working group led by Indigenous researchers, stresses that research must provide immediate tangible benefits to the communities being studied and must help to address inequities and close the many gaps in Indigenous Peoples' health outcomes, by prioritising locally designed and culturally adapted programmes and services, supported by strategies rooted in Indigenous cultures and involving local leadership and decision-making.

The GACD Indigenous Population Working Group presented the view that decolonising and Indigenising research methods and practices are needed to help enable Indigenous Peoples to improve their lives by overcoming the failures of colonial structures, policies, and practices. Furthermore, they encourage decolonising research funding by changing the current practices of awarding grants to a single administering research institution where the principal investigator works, which may then allocate some money to Indigenous institutions. Awarding grants only to external non-indigenous organisations can foster a power imbalance between the researchers and the community, and risks being inequitable. The report of the Working Group concluded by emphasising the need to develop true partnerships and collaborations at all stages of research projects and the importance of recognising the heterogeneity of Indigenous Peoples and their sociocultural, historical, and health contexts.

Many Indigenous groups have high suicide rates. Multiple risk factors are associated with past and present treatment of Indigenous People as marginal or 'second-rate' citizens. Transgenerational traumas, including forced displacement from traditional lands, depriving children of their families and culture by placing them in residential schools, unchecked abuse in residential schools, and restrictive laws have increased vulnerabilities in many Indigenous communities and cultures. Current food and housing insecurities as well as inequities in educational, health care, and other basic services have increased the stresses on Indigenous individuals, families, and communities.

Although the regulations about conducting research with Indigenous Peoples have led to the application of research protocols and collaborations that are of greater benefit to them, suicide prevention research still faces many challenges. Since there are relatively few skilled Indigenous researchers, outside researchers must learn about the Indigenous culture to conduct research in Indigenous communities. Outside researchers often have a bias from what they know of other cultures, which may or may not be pertinent.

Most suicide research on Indigenous populations focuses on risk factors, the negative aspects that increase suicide risk. There is relatively little research focused on protective factors, cultural and community strengths, and traditional coping strategies that have been beneficial. In some instances, large sums of money have been invested in research projects to 'understand' risk factors for suicide in communities where basic needs for food, shelter, jobs, medical care, and recreational activities are sorely lacking. One may question the ethical use of research funds in contexts where the research participants are experiencing inequities and deprivation.

3.11 The Interpretation and Dissemination of Results

There is strong evidence that publicity about death by suicide is associated with an increase in suicides among vulnerable populations who are exposed to that publicity (Mishara and Dargis, 2019; Pirkis *et al.*, 2017; Stack, 2005). What are the positive and negative effects of disseminating the results of suicide research? Consider research findings that identify people who possess certain characteristics as being at greater risk for suicide. Awareness of these results may increase anxiety and concern among groups with such characteristics and could fuel their social stigmatisation. The same effect may be observed when studies show higher suicide risks in particular environments. For example, media reports of a cluster of suicides in a Quebec town resulted in a flurry of sensational reporting on a possible suicide 'epidemic'. A town-wide crisis was created as parents withdrew their children from the local high school. It took more than a year before researchers determined that what seemed to be an epidemic of suicides actually involved unrelated incidents, and that there appeared to be no significant suicide risk factors related to the school environment. Even if there were a greater risk in a specific school, publicising research about this could have the negative effect of increasing anxiety in students and parents without reducing the risk factors themselves (Baker *et al.*, 2021; Mishara, 2003).

Moralists would find themselves forced to evaluate the research findings in order to determine if there were risks of increased suicide associated with disseminating the results. Relativists may compare the potential risks and benefits in terms of potentially saving lives. Libertarians might tend to ignore potential risks and invoke arguments about 'the right to know', and thus might distribute all results, regardless of the consequences.

3.12   Special Issues in Evaluation Research

There are numerous general issues in evaluation research, some of which are not specific to suicidology (Mishara and Tousignant, 2004). Very often, the goals of the evaluation are different from the perspective of those involved. The focus of the evaluation may need to be adjusted, depending on different needs. The goal of evaluators who are outside researchers may be to conduct as scientific an evaluation as possible in order to obtain reliable and valid information, which can be accepted for publication in academic journals. For the board of directors of the local organisation, the goal may be to improve practices. However, the board may have other specific goals, such as justifying the termination of some staff members or obtaining information to assist in funding requests. The director and administration of the agency may be concerned with cost cutting or improving efficiency, or may simply wish to impress on the board of directors that they are doing an exemplary job. Employees might view an evaluation as an opportunity to express their desires to obtain better working conditions. Equally, they could be threatened by the evaluation, since their activities could come under scrutiny.

There are specific ethical issues that arise from conflicts among evaluation objectives. For example, a skilled researcher can develop a client satisfaction questionnaire that is almost certain to obtain positive results, which administrators can use to justify funding requests. In the area of suicide prevention, one is hard-pressed to locate a client satisfaction survey that has not produced extremely positive results. Therefore, the validity and usefulness of client surveys to inform about any specific organisation may be questionable.

Evaluation research may provide data that could assist in making decisions about whether to fund specific programmes. Analyses are often undertaken in which the cost of the activity is weighed against its potential benefits. However, in the area of suicide prevention, how is it possible to measure the value of saving a human life? To a moralist, the importance of saving even one life justifies enormous effort and expense. However, moralists are not supported by unlimited funding and resources. If agencies must choose between funding a very costly programme that is likely to save many lives versus funding a less expensive programme that has the potential to save fewer lives, should the moralist have to accept the programme that saves fewer lives? Libertarians, no matter how much they believe in the choice of suicide, would be expected to encourage making programmes available that allow individuals to freely choose to access help for their problems. Therefore, libertarians may be likely to favour programmes that are responsive to the current needs of clients, rather than more proactive programmes that actively seek to prevent suicide among those who have not asked for help.

Evaluators are faced with the challenge of deciding how to present analyses of the costs and benefits of suicide prevention (Tucker *et al.*, 2019). If their philosophical perspective were more libertarian, there would be a tendency to prioritise variables related to clients' freedom. Moralist-oriented evaluators would look carefully at the potential of programmes to save lives.

Is it possible to prioritise the focus of suicide prevention programmes? If funding is limited, would it be best to finance a programme that has a high potential for saving the lives of elderly suicidal cancer patients or an equally expensive programme having the potential to save fewer lives, but lives of people in the prime of life and in good health? Is it not a safe assumption that most people would respond that it is the latter programme that should be financed? Must we adopt a relativist position that some lives are viewed as more valued and worthier of saving than others? When resources are limited, must moralists then be forced to compromise their values and prioritise which lives are more valued?

Evaluators are faced with these issues in determining not only what type of information to collect in the process of an evaluation, but the type of cost–benefit analyses they may undertake and the manner in which they interpret those findings. For example, many years ago, the Centers for Disease Control and Prevention of the United States, in a conference comparing suicide prevention strategies, said that they were looking for programmes offering 'more bang for the dollar' (Hendin *et al.*, 1985). Such a statement appears to reflect the view that the more lives saved, the better the programme (Ahern *et al.*, 2018; Hendin *et al.*, 1985). However, is there not a moral obligation to also invest in less-efficient programmes to meet the suicide prevention needs of specific subpopulations? For example, even if it were determined to be much less cost-efficient, might it be important to offer more programmes to Indigenous Peoples or other underserved minority groups? Although evaluators pretend to be neutral about such issues, their values and beliefs concerning the rights and obligations of various subgroups of the population are implicit in any evaluation activity.

Confidentiality is usually offered to research participants to make it more likely people will be willing to participate and to ensure that the information obtained is not self-edited for its social desirability, or less biased than if it were not confidential. What is the ethical course of action when, during evaluation research, information is obtained indicating that lives may be inadvertently lost because of poor practices? For example, when conducting a silent monitoring study listening to calls to a helpline where anonymity was promised, what is the researcher's responsibility if the listener hears that some helpers encourage people to kill themselves? Or, more commonly, what if researchers learn that identifiable helpers are not conducting adequate interventions or are interrupting their interventions to take personal calls? While the impact of substandard practices on callers' suicidality may be unknown, researchers' ethics are challenged when incompetence or negligence is revealed to researchers who have promised confidentiality to all participants.

Researchers evaluating clinical interventions face the ethical dilemmas of clinicians: must the information obtained be divulged in order to save the lives of callers, despite promises of confidentiality? This would require retaining identifying information that would otherwise be discarded, disguised, or deleted. The primacy of confidentiality might be tempered by the obligation to provide competent assistance. A cost–benefit analysis of disclosure versus nondisclosure would require estimating the impact of each policy on the quality of evaluation research and the services provided.

One of the important issues in evaluation research is to determine who may use the evaluation results and under what circumstances. In some situations, the evaluation results 'belong' to the researchers, to publish and disseminate as they please. In other situations, the report is submitted to a board of directors, a funding agency, or administrators, who may choose to disseminate all or part of the results as they see fit. It is not unusual that there are conflicts over who has the right to use the evaluation and in what manner. One of the issues facing an evaluator is the extent to which they have an obligation to disseminate the results regardless of what they indicate. (See also the discussion of data ownership in research with Indigenous peoples in the preceding section of this chapter.)

Does the evaluator or researcher have a moral obligation to consider the effects of dissemination of all or part of the results, and to consider the manner in which the results are interpreted? Very often the way results are presented depends on how the evaluators view the findings. For example, an ethical dilemma may occur when the evaluation of a community's only suicide prevention programme indicates that there are some serious deficiencies. If this information is disseminated, clients may stop seeking help at that agency because they feel they will not get good service. They may not sufficiently comprehend that, despite the deficiencies, there is still a net value in continued consultation. Community politicians motivated to cut spending may interpret the evaluation results as a reason to set suicide prevention aside rather than improve services. This points to the fact that evaluation data, like all research data, are not simple facts. The way in which they are presented and interpreted may have an important influence on practices, and eventually on the saving of lives.

Would a moralist condone downplaying negative results so that an organisation could continue functioning and helping prevent suicides? Otherwise, accurate dissemination of results, which could result in limiting services, might ultimately save more lives by bringing about better suicide prevention practises. Would the libertarian perspective suggest that research results should be disseminated in as neutral a manner as possible, without any further deliberations or calculations? The relativist might examine the specific situation, but it may not be at all clear which variables take precedence for effective policymaking, regardless of any pre-existing hierarchy of social values.

3.13   New Technologies, Artificial Intelligence, and Moral Redefinition

3.13.1   Informed Consent and Confidentiality

As more suicide prevention activities are occurring over the Internet, using online programs and text or chat exchanges from smartphones, there is a rapidly increasing body of research studying online behaviours in relation to suicide and using artificial intelligence (AI) to develop algorithms for the detection and prediction of suicidal behaviours. There has been much public attention to the issues concerning confidentiality of digital information and activities, as well as to the challenges of obtaining informed consent for conducting research on personal data that are either publicly available or have been collected by profit-making companies (e.g., Google, Amazon, Facebook, Instagram). When users click on 'I accept' to use or install a program, they usually accept a blanket statement that the service providers and software manufacturers can do pretty much anything they please with private data. This acceptance is used to justify using or selling personal data to add to the provider's profits. Legally, consumers attest to the fact that they have 'read' and 'understood' what they were signing. The fact that they rarely read the contracts they sign may not absolve consumers from having given away the rights to their information. However, this practice is ethically challenging, particularly since consumers are not provided with the option of refusing to 'accept' the terms, whatever they may be, if they want to use the program, access social media, or use other services. It is possible that future legislation may offer consumers more protection and the right to avoid unwanted use of their digital data and information on their online activity. In the absence of robust protective legislation, private companies can set their own ethical standards and are not obliged to follow national or international ethical guidelines.

In contrast, researchers in most countries are bound to strict ethical guidelines for their activities and use of personal information. Professional organisations, institutional affiliations, and funding agencies concur that research involving human subjects must be approved by an institutional Research Ethics Board Committee. Among other requirements, researchers must follow the rule of informed consent. This requires researchers to obtain approval from individuals whose data they want to study and inform people about why and how their information will be used. This requirement may compel researchers from using data that are regularly exploited for profit by corporate entities, and data which may be openly accessible to the general public.

Obtaining informed consent is complicated by the quasi-anonymity offered by the Internet. The issues of rescue procedures we discussed in the beginning of this chapter become more challenging when users do not identify themselves. Without contact information, it may be practically impossible to trace a person's location or identity. Furthermore, as the abilities of hackers continually keep pace with technologies designed to protect anonymity and sensitive personal information, the ability to guarantee privacy to research participants may diminish.

In the future, are we destined to abandon privacy as we now know it, replacing it with a culture that is continually trying to develop encryption programs to hang on to some personal information we hold dear, against the tide of hacking tools to investigate everything about us? If our suicidal behaviours, thoughts, and intentions are to be revealed to the world, will citizens be left with damaging consequences? For the optimists, the ability to analyse big data sets to identify people at risk and intervene should result in a future world where more suicides are prevented. Potentially, all suicidality would thus be identified and most suicides prevented, assuming also that more effective suicide prevention methods will be perfected. The ethical quandary involves balancing concerns for the ability to maintain privacy and autonomy against the moral obligations to help and protect vulnerable people.

Some companies are likely to develop ways of monetising the analysis of the suicide risk of individuals, using increasingly reliable AI-generated methods. If there are financial incentives to actively engage in suicide prevention, for example by increasing the reputation of the company as being benevolent, might this foster disregard for privacy issues? However, if the financial benefits appear greater when strict privacy is respected, could this inhibit suicide prevention? If a for-profit suicide prevention organisation pays to have suicidal people referred to them, are there ethical considerations that are different from the suggestions to use paid advertisers when we are looking to buy a product?

3.13.2   Risk Prediction and Equity Issues

In suicidology, most of the current use of new technologies is to identify and predict people at risk of suicide. The use of these automated technologies, including sophisticated AI programs, can lead to hidden biases, which can create ethical challenges concerning equity. Algorithms created by AI can identify people at elevated suicide risk. These programs are being used to screen people accessing suicide prevention services. For example, a suicide prevention chat service may receive far more requests for chat help than it is able to provide. It may then decide that it wants to give priority to people who are the most likely to be at risk of attempting suicide and may develop a screening questionnaire to assess who should get the timeliest access to the chat services, with the understanding that some 'low risk' people may never be able to access the service.

This analysis would then be used to move higher-risk people to the top of the wait list to obtain quicker access to help. Men are generally four or more times at risk of killing themselves than women, in most countries. An intelligent program whose goal is to identify as many at-risk people as possible and provide priority services to them could ensure that men always get priority over women, other important risk factors being equal. This could result in almost all the men getting help and a majority of women not being able to access the service. Can this practise be considered equitable?

Should women have a right to a certain 'equitable' proportion of services, even if men have a statistically much higher probability of dying by suicide? Women often have much higher rates of nonlethal suicide attempts. Is it ethically justified to focus on saving lives as a priority over preventing suicide attempts? These questions parallel ethical debates in medicine over what proportion of the medical services budget should be devoted to preventing the development of illnesses such as diabetes or cancer and what proportion should be spent on treating people who are already acutely ill. In an ideal world, one should do both, and everyone who seeks help from a suicide prevention service should get it. However, resources for suicide prevention are often insufficient, and decisions about what constitutes ethical and equitable access must be made. If computer programs are being used to screen for risk, they need to be designed to ensure that access to services is equitable, in the manner determined to be ethical by the service providers.

3.13.3 Future Technology and Moral Redefinition

In the future, the transition from seeking help by direct human contact to the use of digital technologies to solve all manner of human dilemmas will accelerate exponentially as AI begets computer programs capable of constantly improving their accuracy and efficiency in attaining the goals they are programmed to achieve. Suicide prevention will no longer involve what the founder of modern suicide prevention, Edwin Shneidman (1973, p. xiii) felt was the essence of interventions to prevent people from killing themselves: 'meaningful (and often stressful) dyadic relationships'. Help provided or brokered by autonomous self-improving AI programs using machine-learning technologies will likely be omnipresent in suicide prevention. Constantly evolving and self-perfecting algorithms will be used to rapidly assess suicide risk in ways that are so complex that their nature will surpass human understanding. Therapy bots that have what seem to be unlimited capacities, require no salary, have low maintenance, and never fatigue or experience burnout will become the norm. Clinical decisions, such as when to hospitalise an at-risk person against the person's will, will be determined automatically by algorithms in programs that learn from their experiences.

Stephen Hawking expressed concerns that AI could evolve over time to attain its goals amorally, albeit lacking in malice. He used an analogy: 'You are probably not an evil ant-hater who steps on ants out of malice, but if you're in charge of a hydroelectric green energy project and there's an anthill in the region to be flooded, too bad for the ants. Let's not place humanity in the position of those ants' (Hawking, 2015). He also said:

> As emphasised by Steve Omohundro, an extremely intelligent future AI will probably develop a drive to survive and acquire more resources as a step toward accomplishing whatever goal it has, because surviving and having more resources will increase its chances of accomplishing that other goal. This can cause problems for humans whose resources get taken away.

Assuming that the human race will find ways of taming resource-hungry AI programs, suicide prevention will face the ethical challenge of ensuring equity when programs focus on augmenting success, accuracy, and efficiency. We have already seen this equity issue play out when AI programs are used to analyse questionnaire responses to privilege access to suicide prevention chat interventions by systematically choosing men over women. People with complex severe mental health problems who have lower 'success' rates in response to treatments could similarly be given low priority in order to improve the efficient use of resources. An important challenge is for suicide prevention to find the means to ensure that all suicidal individuals have equitable access to help, in an age where the quantity of people helped and efficiency in the use of resources may be the normative goals.

3.13.4   An Ethical Checklist for the Use of Artificial Intelligence in Suicide Prevention

It is rare that research publications that report on the use of AI in suicide prevention include a discussion of ethical concerns or challenges. One way to encourage increased attention to ethical aspects of AI in research is to provide a detailed checklist that describes the primary ethical considerations in research and practice. Mörch *et al.* (2020) developed what they believe to be the first AI checklist in this field, the Canada Protocol, a checklist for the use of AI in suicide prevention and mental health. The Canada Protocol is based on a systematic literature review of documents discussing ethical challenges in the use of AI in suicide research, suicide prevention, and mental health. A first version was refined and validated by a Delphi consultation with stakeholders and experts. Their final checklist contains thirty-eight items of potential ethical concerns, divided into five categories: Description (of the project and methods), Privacy and Transparency, Security, Health-Related Risks, and Biases. Each item is formulated to explore an area of ethical concern and requests information to address the concerns. For example:

– In the project's Description section, one of the eight items is 'Evidence', which says: 'If you made claims about your Autonomous Intelligent System's efficacy, performance, or benefits, please justify them and provide the evidence underlying them. If you have mentioned or used scientific papers, please cite your sources.'

- Under Privacy and Transparency, the item 'Right to be forgotten' asks: 'Describe whether an individual can retrieve and erase all of his or her information, and if so, how. Describe the mechanism.'
- An example under Security is 'Data protection': 'Detail all the measures taken to protect any sensitive and personal information.'
- Under Health-Related Risks, one of the items asks about 'Crisis and contingency planning': 'List the criteria for evaluating the risk exposure of your Autonomous Intelligent System. Describe your plan in case of emergency, disaster, or suicidal crisis (the intervention protocol). If possible, specify what type of behaviours and environments are considered as being at risk and explain the rationale in a simple way.'
- An example in the category of Biases, 'Stigmatisation,' states: 'Describe how you avoided using languages, images, and other content that could stigmatise users (e.g., reference guidelines on safe media reporting and public messaging about suicide and mental illness).'

The authors of the Canada Protocol admit that ethical tools such as this checklist are not sufficient to ensure that AI is used ethically. They note that legal systems must be updated to address new and emerging ethical challenges, and institutions and organisations need to provide more ethical guidance to AI developers, starting in the early stage of their projects. Furthermore, Institutional Research Ethics Boards need to include members with expertise in AI and in the ethical challenges of using digital technologies.

3.14   Conclusions and Recommendations

The examples in this chapter illustrate the extent to which ethical considerations influence decisions by researchers in the design, conduct, and dissemination of their studies. Although our ethical perspectives of the moralist, libertarian, and relativist are useful in understanding how decisions can be and have been made, it is evident that having a clearly defined moral stance is not, in and of itself, sufficient to determine what to do when faced with important ethical dilemmas in suicidology research. The reality of conducting research may require a mix of ethical perspectives and the development of a pragmatic approach, which is more complicated than choosing one philosophical perspective.

The strict moralist is induced to evaluate whose lives are more valued if there are insufficient resources. In reality, few moralists would invest as much to save the life of a condemned serial killer as opposed to a productive citizen. Libertarians may claim to be neutral concerning the right to live and die, leaving it to everyone's personal discretion. However, part of the concept of liberty to choose involves the liberty to seek help. Is there not an implied understanding on the part of the libertarians to help individuals express choice through seeking help based on quality services? Libertarians are also confronted with the challenges of special populations who may be considered incompetent to exercise their free choice, or may be under pressure to choose to live or die. For example, if a person chooses to die because of intolerable pain and suffering in a society where pain control is not an acceptable practice, is this a free choice? In a cult where the leader has brainwashed members into following his every whim, if the leader orders people to kill themselves, do the members freely choose to die? Is freedom to choose to die extended to minors, or are there parental obligations to save their lives? Relativists may accommodate certain situations where intervention is obligatory or where people should be left to decide. In situations where we do not have sufficient knowledge to determine if the circumstances meet their criteria, might it be best to try to save everyone and slide towards a moralist position, or rather let each person be free to choose, as a libertarian would espouse?

One of the ways by which researchers may avoid some of the pitfalls of ethical challenges is to clarify in advance their moral stance concerning suicide and its implications for their research. It is possible to set out the ethical values that are to govern the research in a description of the research project, in the research proposal, or in a contract to conduct an evaluation study. We suggest that the statement of values may begin with a position concerning the morality of suicide and the ethics of prevention and intervention. The researchers may then elaborate on relevant aspects of their activities involving ethical issues, stating in specific terms how some of these issues will be handled and how they will be resolved.

Such a document could include a statement of whether confidential information will ever be disclosed, and if so to whom, in what manner, and under what circumstances. Rescue procedures for participants may be described, including the criteria to be employed for rescue as well as the nature of the rescue activities that are to be made available. This may also have a description of to whom the results will be communicated, who may use the results, and in what manner. Finally, researchers may state what will occur if negative findings are obtained, or if situations arise that may increase the probability of suicide, either indirectly or directly.

This chapter has explored how ethical presuppositions concerning suicide influence research practises. It is our hope this will stimulate further discussion of the relationships between ethical and legal positions, and their implications for research. Consideration of these issues may avoid potentially difficult situations that could negatively affect investigations. The handling of these ethical issues will inevitably impact the lives of suicidal people who are involved in the research as well as those who could benefit from the results. In the future, as automated programs using AI increasingly replace human decision-making and interventions, we will face more ethical challenges concerning respect for autonomy and privacy as well as concerns for equitable use of resources. As Stephen Hawking pleaded, we must learn to think not only about how to create AI, but also about how to ensure its beneficial use. As the field of suicide prevention increasingly embraces the use of AI, we must remain steadfast in linking calculations of benefits and losses to reflective ethical considerations.

4

• • • • • • •

The Control of Suicide Promotion over the Internet

There has been growing concern about the numerous reports of suicides and suicidal behaviours following contact with websites that incite people to suicide and provide detailed information on suicide methods, as well as exposing people to online suicide content (Alao *et al.*, 2006; Australian IT, 2004; Baeva, 2020; Baume *et al.*, 1997; Becker and Schmidt, 2004; Dobson, 1999; Mehlum, 2000; Paul *et al.*, 2017; Rajagopal, 2004; Reuter, 2004; Richard *et al.*, 2000; Totaro *et al.*, 2016). This phenomenon has inspired efforts to make the encouragement of suicide over the Internet illegal (e.g., Bychkova and Radnayeva, 2018; Phillips *et al.*, 2019; Rimmer, 2019; Taylor, 2019; Yaremko and Banakh, 2018). Surveys of the content of websites accessed by young people seeking information about suicide on the Internet found that 16% of sites provide specific advice on how to harm oneself and 7% encouraged self-harm (Singaravelu *et al.*, 2015). This chapter, which updates Mishara & Weisstub, (2007) focuses on the ethical, legal, and practical issues in the control and regulation of suicide promotion and assistance over the Internet.

4.1 Media Reports on Internet Encouragement of Suicide

In December 2021, the *New York Times* published a detailed investigative report on a website started in 2018 that encouraged people to kill themselves and provided detailed instructions and information on how to kill oneself (Twohey and Dance, 2021). The report documented that over 500 members, more than two a week, wrote 'goodbye threads' in which members indicated how and when they planned to end their lives. Some described their ongoing suicide in real time or live-streamed their deaths as others watched. The report identified at least 45 people who died by suicide in the United States (USA), Canada, the United Kingdom (UK), and Australia.

Multiple suicides by people who meet on chat sites appear to be increasing. One much-publicised early example concerned Louis Gillies from Glasgow, who met Michael Gooden from East Sussex (England) in May 2002 on a suicide 'newsgroup' (Innes, 2003). While on a cliff ready to jump, Gillies was talked out of killing himself by a friend speaking on his mobile phone, but Gooden refused to talk and jumped. Gillies was charged with aiding and abetting a suicide. Gillies killed himself in April 2003, just before his trial was about to begin. In Japan, the phenomenon in which people exchange suggestions about suicide and make suicide pacts is called *netto shinju*. Ikunaga *et al.* (2013) conducted a systematic analysis of popular Japanese suicide bulletin boards and found that 12% of the discussions were about suicide pacts. Lee and Kwon (2018) observed that social media in Japan such as Twitter (now X) frequently contain potentially 'dangerous' content. Each year, scientific journals have published case studies of suicide pacts where people met on the Internet (e.g., Tusiewicz *et al.*, 2022).

Meeting suicide companions online appears to be most prevalent in Japan, where the trend started over 20 years ago. Between February and early June 2003, at least 20 Japanese died in suicide pacts with companions they met on the Internet, many by strikingly similar carbon monoxide poisonings (Harding, 2004). This increased to 60 deaths in suicide pacts by 2007 (Naito, 2007). In mainland China, 159 suicide pact deaths from 62 different pacts were reported (Jiang *et al.*, 2017). It is believed that in South Korea the first wave of internet suicide pacts occurred in 2000, when there were three cases. In March 2003, an Austrian teenager and a 40-year-old Italian who met on a suicide chat room jointly died by suicide near Vienna (Mishara and Weisstub, 2007). The man had also contacted two young Germans online, but police alerted their families before they could carry out their suicides. Cheng (2011) suggested that internet service providers could be held responsible for online suicide pacts, since they have permitted posts in which users seek someone to carry out a suicide with them.

4.2   Legal Provisions and Law Reform Projects

Many countries have laws prohibiting the aiding and abetting of suicide (see Chapter 7 for a list of laws by country). On 13 February 2005, Gerald Krein was arrested in Oregon for solicitation to commit murder after it was alleged that he used his internet chat room to entice up to 31 lonely single women to kill themselves on Valentine's Day (Booth, 2005). The arrest followed a report to police by a woman in the chat room who said another participant talked about killing her two children before taking her own life (Booth, 2005).

Why then have current laws against aiding and abetting suicide not been applied to internet activities, given the compelling nature of specific case histories in which people died by suicide in a manner communicated over the Internet, following a series of internet contacts in which they were encouraged to kill themselves? The high incidence of internet-related suicides in Japan has resulted in the publication of numerous calls for legislative reform (Hensel, 2020; Phillips *et al.*, 2019).

In order to understand the lack of legislation addressing this issue, it is helpful to examine jurisprudence regarding standards for determining causality in such matters. When individuals are deemed to be responsible for having caused harm to another person, their actions are usually in close temporal and physical proximity to the victim and the victim's death. In addition, scientific and medical evidence must indicate, according to reasonable probabilities, that the action in question was causally related to the consequences (Bongar, 2002).

Scientific research on the influence of the media on suicides has concentrated on television and newspapers and their influence on population suicide rates. There are several excellent reviews of research in this area (e.g., Hawton and Williams, 2001; Pirkis, 2019; Pirkis *et al.*, 2014; Stack, 2003, 2005). It is clear that news media depictions of deaths by suicide have the risk of increasing suicides among those who have contact with those media. Generally, the more publicity, the higher the contagion effect. It has been estimated that the suicide of Marilyn Monroe resulted in 197 additional suicides (Phillips, 1974). However, there are no empirical data on changes in the risk of suicide that may be related to contact with internet sites. Nevertheless, it appears from numerous cases reported in the media that contact with internet sites and with chat rooms preceded some deaths by suicide and that the methods used were precisely those described in the internet contact. In sum, these case reports do not meet the requirements for scientific proof that internet sites cause suicide, but they suggest that a relationship may exist.

Despite the case reports that suggest an association, it can be argued that, had the victims not contacted a specific suicide site, they still might have killed themselves. The suicide risk of people who contact suicide sites may have pre-dated their contact, possibly prompting them to conduct a search for the sites or make contact on the sites. In addition, if a person had not used the method found on a site, other methods were easily available.

Another challenge in determining a causal relationship is the difficulty in generalising from epidemiological population statistics to individual cases. According to population statistics, it has been demonstrated that media publicity on suicide results in a small but significant increase in the number of people who die by suicide following the media reports. It is not possible, however, to generalise from these population data to determine if any one specific individual's death was facilitated by their having read a newspaper article or having watched a specific television programme about suicide. The population-level data, given the great number of people at risk of attempting suicide and the very small number who actually • die by suicide, do not permit researchers to determine that one specific individual is likely to have died as a result of media exposure and that the death could have been avoided by nonexposure. To date, we have only a small number of anecdotal case histories in which there appears to be a link. Without further research data, one cannot make a solid scientific or legal argument for the causal relationship between internet activities and suicide.

4.2.1 Self-regulation

In most countries, there is little or no control of internet content because of constitutional guarantees of freedom of expression and a reluctance to regulate speech. This may conflict with attempts to prevent suicide or regulate access to sites that promote suicide. European Union (EU) decision number 276–1999, 'The European Union Safer Internet Plan' (European Union, 1999), essentially proposes that internet organisations and internet service providers (ISPs) act responsibly to control what is available and limit or deny access to sites that are illegal or dangerous. Many countries, including Great Britain, Canada, the USA, and New Zealand, attempt to control internet content by self-regulation, since guarantees of freedom of speech apparently preclude censorship or government control of access to sites. As has been seen, self-regulation generally fails to limit what is available on the Internet, and the libertarian approach of many technology firms suggests little will change in this regard. Additionally, there is little agreement as to what content should or must be banned, and few legal mechanisms to enforce such bans.

4.2.2 Filtering Techniques

An alternative to self-regulation is a rating system that uses filtering techniques to block access to certain sites installed on personal computers, for instance, parental controls, which allow parents to set filters for what their children can access. Software used to filter sites by blocking access is only effective if it is used, if it blocks target sites, and if it does not block other permissible sites. A primary issue is who actually rates the sites so that filter programs can identify which sites to block. The World Wide Web Consortium (W3C) developed the Platform for Internet Content Selection (PICS) standards (Swick, 2005), in which creators of sites rate their own sites according to specific criteria. This web platform and its successor are no longer maintained since they have been considered to be problematic and ineffective. The filters that have been developed to date have had limited success in discriminating between desirable and undesirable sites. Thus, if filters block access to certain words or topics, for example 'suicide methods', they may also block sites that provide helpful information on suicide prevention, such as the site of Befrienders Worldwide, which offers information and help over the Internet to suicidal individuals (www.befrienders.org).

4.2.3   Blocking Access to Sites

Social media, search engines, and chatbots today generally have software firewalls to block access to content that is illegal. A variety of countries, including Algeria, Bahrain, China, Germany, Iran, North Korea, Saudi Arabia, Singapore, South Korea, Sweden, the United Arab Emirates, and Vietnam, have passed legislation or have the practice of requiring internet service providers to block all access to specific internet sites. For example, in Saudi Arabia all 30 of the ISPs go through a central node, and material and sites containing pornography, material believed to cause religious offence, and information on bomb-making are blocked. Germany requires ISPs to block media that are morally harmful to youth, including those that are pornographic or depict extreme violence or warmongering, or have racist, fascist, or anti-Semitic content. They have had success in blocking German sites with this material but have been less successful in blocking sites originating outside of Germany. Sweden has laws that require blocking of information instigating rebellion, racial agitation, child pornography, illegal description of violence, and material that infringes on copyright laws. In several countries, including the USA, Great Britain, and New Zealand, laws were passed to block certain internet content, but those laws were overturned by the courts because of constitutional guarantees of freedom of expression.

Australia is the only country that currently has laws to specifically restrict sites that promote suicide or provide information on suicide methods (Commonwealth of Australia, 2005). Public concern about the vulnerability of Australian youth gave rise to the enactment of amendments to the Australian federal criminal code, making intentional internet activity relating directly or indirectly to the incitement of suicide a distinct crime (Commonwealth of Australia, 2005). The Australian legislation also bars promotion of particular methods of suicide or providing instruction in them.

The parliamentary debate highlighted the vulnerability of young adults as a particular group, based on both their level of internet usage and their suicide rates (Commonwealth of Australia, 2005). It was argued that because of those factors there is a moral obligation on the part of society to provide protection. The legislators cited the failure of private ISPs to regulate themselves, thereby mandating government to do so. While acknowledging the division in public opinion, the Australian government argued that public protection trumped issues of liberty and freedom of expression.

There was strong vocal opposition, including from the Greens Party. The critics said that the ambiguity of 'intentionality' in the Australian criminal code could have unintended results and could render the law impossible to apply. The point was argued that, given the volume of suicide items incorporated into daily activity on the Internet, it could be foreseen that ISPs could readily find themselves vulnerable to the legislation despite their efforts to control content, if an aggressive pattern of verifications would take place. It was suggested that attacking the causes of suicide, rather than operating with a wide net of surveillance and intervention, would be more likely to succeed in reducing the threat.

Other criticisms addressed the foolhardiness of attempting to restrict information about matters such as suicide and voluntary euthanasia. The key issue, from the point of view of the opposition, was not the need to control internet content, but the extent to which the government was prepared to devote resources to suicide prevention activities.

Five years after the Australian law banning pro-suicide websites was adopted, Pirkis *et al.* (2009) described a continuing 'heated' debate in Australian society. Opponents of the law contended that the law cast too wide a net in its ban of internet content, it interfered with the autonomy of those who wish to die, and, because of jurisdictional enforcement limitations, it had no effect on offshore sites that were accessible from Australia. Proponents of the law found it beneficial to limit access to domestic pro-suicide sites and felt that the law increased awareness of suicide in the community and served as an expression of societal social norms that condemned the promotion of suicidal behaviour.

In 2012, Russia modified its law 'On Protection of Children from Information Harmful to Their Health and Development' to ban sites that disseminate 'dangerous' content, including content that incites suicide and content that contains 'suicide instructions' (Maida, 2017), as Australia had done. Some contend that this law has been used to censure political content not related to suicide that does not pose a danger to children (Maida, 2017).

In 2018, the Ukraine modified its 2007 law condemning incitation to attempt suicide (Yaremko and Banakh, 2018). The original law recognised the crime of incitation to attempt suicide only in the following contexts: (1) Cruel treatment; (2) Blackmail; (3) Coercion for unlawful actions; or (4) the systematic humiliation of human dignity. In 2018 the Ukraine expanded the third and fourth criteria to systematic humiliation of dignity or systemic unlawful coercion of actions that are contrary to the person's will, predilection for suicide, as well as other actions that contribute to suicide. These modifications allow for a broad interpretation of what constitutes incitation to or aiding in suicide. They were enacted to facilitate criminal prosecution for online incitation to suicide, in reaction to what was perceived at the time to be an increase in suicides that the media associated with internet communications among youths inciting others to kill themselves.

4.3   Ethical Presuppositions

There are several ethical considerations concerning the control of internet content to prevent suicide. Those who adopt a libertarian perspective (see Chapter 1) might contend that people have the right to choose to end their life by suicide. Also, since suicide is not illegal in most countries, one could argue that suicidal people should have access to whatever suicide content they desire. If this libertarian position is adopted, it is not possible to justify controlling access to information encouraging suicide, or to control the provision of information or advice on how to exercise the right to end one's life by suicide.

If one adopts a moralist ethical position that suicide must always be prevented, and if controlling access to internet sites can save lives, then controls must be instituted. If one holds a relativist position that some suicides are acceptable and others are not, one may morally justify some form of internet control, although controlling access for only some people is practically impossible. For example, a relativist who believes that terminally ill people should be allowed to have access to means to end their lives, but people in good health who suffer from treatable psychiatric problems should not, would find it impossible to control access for some people and not others.

4.3.1   The Internet Versus Other Mass Media

One of the questions concerning the ethics of controlling access to the Internet is the specificity of the Internet compared with other mass media. The Internet has been characterised as a 'pull' technology, as opposed to the so-called 'push' technologies, including radio and television. Push technologies provide access to the media without the user engaging in any specific and explicit attempt to find a specific media content. Television content is available in every home, and because of its universal access, television has been regulated in most countries as to content. In contrast to the mass media of television and radio, internet users must actively seek out a specific content.

Also, anonymity of the provider can exist on the Internet, and it may be substantially more difficult to verify the authenticity of the information one finds on a website. Thus far, no government agencies are ensuring that Web content is appropriate and accurate (unlike television and radio, which are generally subject to government control). The Web can be extremely graphic in nature, and individuals who display their suicidal intentions and behaviours on the Internet can expect possible exposure to thousands throughout the world, providing glorification of their suicidal acts.

The differences between 'push' and 'pull' technologies may be used to defend the Internet against control by claiming that the Internet is a private service that does not invade people's homes, and that specific content must be sought out by individuals actively searching through cyberspace. The downside, of course, is that this same private status provides for a level of anonymity of both the person contacting the site and the person providing information on a site, which may lead to an 'anything goes' environment where there are no controls whatsoever about the authenticity and credibility of information transmitted or provided.

In addition to websites, people engage with others on the Internet in chat rooms and forums, which can be entirely unregulated. Such forums and chats may draw people in without explicitly describing themselves as focused on a topic. For instance, a person might post a question about suicide in a forum and receive detailed responses or end up in direct communication. This type of internet activity has been nearly impossible to regulate.

4.3.2   Different Internet Activities

Internet situations involving suicide vary. Some sites passively provide information that encourages suicide in texts that suggest it is a good idea to end one's life. Other sites provide information on suicide methods, and many include specific details about what medications to mix, how to hang oneself, and the strengths and weaknesses of alternative methods with respect to side effects and risks of failure. Still other sites involve the exchange of messages from 'suicide encouragers' who interact with suicidal people, trying to stimulate them to proceed with their suicidal plans in chat rooms or in email correspondence. 'Suicide predators' seek out people who post messages that suggest they may be feeling suicidal but who are not explicitly asking for information or encouragement. These predators offer unsolicited incitation to suicide and may provide information about how to carry out suicide without being asked. If one is considering some form of control of internet activity, it is important to decide which of the above activities one would like to limit.

4.3.3   Vulnerable Populations

One of the major issues in control of the Internet to prevent suicides is the protection of minors and other vulnerable populations, such as people with psychiatric disorders. Thus far, very little has been done to protect minors from suicide promotion sites. In the area of the exposure of minors to extreme violence on the Internet, research has shown that media exposure to violence is related to increased violent behaviour (Bushman and Anderson, 2001; Scharrer, 2015); however, there has been little success in attempts to control violence on the Internet.

4.3.4   The Jurisdictional Challenge

Even if one were able to resolve the legal and ethical issues, there are several practical considerations that make control of internet suicide promotion activities extremely difficult (Geist, 2002; Mishara and Weisstub, 2007; Rimmer, 2019; Smith, 2002). The first is the issue of cross-border jurisdiction. Although countries may be able to control activities of internet sites that originate within their borders, international jurisprudence makes it difficult to obtain jurisdiction over sites that originate outside the country. Jurisprudence generally distinguishes between passive internet activity, such as simply operating a website that may be accessed from different countries, and active endeavours, which involve sending information, interacting (e.g., in a chat room), and doing business in a country. Furthermore, jurisprudence has favoured limiting claims of harm to actual impact rather than claims of potential damage.

Two important cases underline the difficulties in cross-border jurisdiction issues. The first case in Canada, *Braintech, Inc. v. Kostiuk* (1999), involved a libel complaint concerning a site originating or hosted in Canada. In denying jurisdiction, the judge found that there is a 'need for better proof the defendant entered Texas than the mere possibility that someone in Texas may have reached to cyberspace to bring defamation material to a screen in Texas'. The ability to access material from an internet site hosted outside a given jurisdiction from within that jurisdiction was not sufficient to allow for regulation by entities outside that jurisdiction (Geist, 2002).

The Calder test, based on the US case of *Calder v. Jones* (1984), is often used to determine jurisdiction in internet cases. This test requires that the defendant's intentional tortuous actions: (1) are expressly aimed at the forum state and (2) cause harm to the plaintiff in the forum state, which the defendant knows is likely to be suffered. This test provides protection for internet sites and activities that do not explicitly attempt to have an effect outside of their own jurisdiction or intentionally cause harm to an individual in another jurisdiction. Certainly, it is both wise and practical to protect individuals from being liable in every country in the world for actions that may be perfectly legal in their own jurisdiction. Still, jurisdiction issues make attempts to control internet activity extremely difficult.

4.4 Suicide and the Darknet

So far our discussion in this chapter has concerned internet content that is considered to be public, information that is accessible by conventional search engines such as Google. The Internet also contains private content that is only accessible to users who install specific software, such as Tor ('The Onion Router'), referred to as the Darknet or the 'Deep Web'. This software makes it almost impossible to identify the users. The Darknet is therefore a host to various illegal activities such as the sale of drugs and illegal weapons, and access to illegal pornographic content. Although there has been much research on suicide content available on the public Surface Web, there has been much less research and discussion of the suicide content on the Darknet. Because of their secret private content, sites and information on the Darknet are not referenced or indexed, and their content, the software used to access the Darknet, circumvents attempts at censorship because of the relative anonymity of users and avoids restrictions imposed on search engines by government regulators. Therefore, the discussions about control of access to internet content do not apply to the Darknet.

Mörch *et al.* (2018) published the first investigation of the nature and accessibility of suicide-related information available on the Darknet, using nine different search engines designed to access the Darknet. They searched for 'suicide' and 'suicide method' and identified 476 sites, with very few (4%) specifically dedicated to the topic of suicide. Over half the sites were not accessible or did not contain suicide content. However, they identified several forums ('chat boards') where suicide was a topic. These sites usually had content encouraging suicide and discussing suicide methods, and access to the sites was blocked in Surface Web search engines.

The presence of suicide content on the Darknet is important to consider in the context of any discussion of controlling access to content on the public Surface Web. The Darknet's presence indicates that, regardless of attempts to control access to suicide content by search engines, social media, or government legislation, any suicide content imaginable can exist on the Darknet and can be accessible to anyone who installs one of the free Darknet search engines that are readily available. The authors of this study suggest that Darknet content needs further study and must be considered when developing suicide prevention strategies for internet content.

4.5   Conclusions

There remains a great need for scientifically valid data on the extent to which exposure to and/or participation on pro-suicide internet sites contributes to the risk of suicide. Before developing national or international standards to protect the public from dangerous pro-suicide sites, we need to determine if specific internet activities increase suicide risk and, if so, which subpopulations are particularly vulnerable. Sensational media reports of suicides following internet activities, and dramatic case reports of individuals who died by suicide using methods they found on the Internet or in pacts with people they met over the Internet, do not constitute scientific proof that internet activities provoke suicides. One could investigate the relationship between internet activities and suicide using psychological autopsy methods. Qualitative assessments of the content of internet contacts where seemingly vulnerable individuals appear to have been forcefully encouraged to kill themselves have high face validity, that is, they appear so to most observers. However, we need to develop more creative methodologies, perhaps inspired by the studies of the relationship between suicide reporting in other media and suicide rates. One of the greatest challenges is to determine the likelihood that individuals who kill themselves after internet contacts would have died by suicide if they had not used the Internet.

It is also important to clarify the ethical basis on which any form of suicide prevention activity is undertaken before applying one's beliefs to controlling internet suicide promotion. Furthermore, any action to control internet suicide promotion must consider the different forms of internet activities, which range from passive posting of information on a website, to interacting in a chat room, to seeking out vulnerable individuals as an internet predator.

Any attempt to control the Internet must be viewed along with the control and freedom of other media, unless special characteristics of the Internet are judged to lead to special laws or consideration. It can be argued that the Internet lacks quality control, and this may justify legislative intervention. We must keep in mind, however, that editors of newspapers, like webmasters, are free to publish what they please, even if it may incite suicides. If a journalist publishes a 'dangerous' article, they may invoke the ire of readers and sales may decline (or increase due to the controversy). When a website or chat does something people do not like, users can simply not frequent that site. In this regard it is interesting to compare the Internet to published works. If one were to publish the philosopher David Hume's writings recommending suicide on an Australian internet site, would this be banned? If so, would it be considered more dangerous than publishing his book and selling it in a bookstore? Internet sites provide information on means to kill oneself in an often clear but informal manner. However, if the same information is available in medical textbooks, what would justify control of this information over the Internet while the sale of medical textbooks and their availability in libraries are permitted?

The fact that the Internet allows for global access leads to complex jurisdictional issues and practical difficulties. Given the rapidly changing state of technology, which has continually led to the rapid development of new ways to circumvent control, it may not be feasible to ban sites, censor material, or limit access. Even if data to document that high risks of suicide are related to specific internet activities were available, and even if a country decides to prevent access to pro-suicide sites, the only way to ensure even a minimal level of success would be to install draconian censorship measures. Since the likelihood of effective control of access to pro-suicide material is not certain to be effective, alternatives to control and censorship should be considered, such as developing and disseminating increased suicide prevention activities on the Internet to counteract internet suicide promotion activities. Persons trained in suicide prevention could be deployed to enter chat discussions to dissuade suicidal people from killing themselves and encourage them to seek help. Finally, public education could be enhanced to facilitate access to ways and means to obtain help from the Internet in the interest of suicide prevention.

5
• • • • • • •

Genetic Testing for Suicide Risk Assessment

Over the past fifty years, geneticists and neuroscientists have been rushing to locate the biological bases of human behaviours. Such evidence, they claim, would change our notions about freedom of choice and enter the universe of determinism based on biomarkers and other salient physiological indicators. In the area of suicide, genetic markers have been sought with the hope that evidence might be located in the genome that predicts who will attempt suicide. The impetus was originally to create genetic profiles so that we could arrive at a genetic parallel with medical conditions such as Huntington's disease and some forms of cancer, which would identify clear indicators of the risk of a future suicide. From such information, individuals who carried the genetic risk could be targeted for prevention measures. There has been optimistic speculation. For example, an article in the *MIT Technology Review* stated, 'While claims for a suicide test remain preliminary, and controversial, a "suicide gene" is not as fanciful as it sounds. The chance that a person takes his or her own life is in fact heritable, and many scientific teams are now involved in broad expeditions across the human genome to locate suicide's biological causes' (Regalado, 2014). This chapter explores the ethical premises and practical challenges underlying the clinical use of genetic testing in predicting suicide risk, based upon the review by Mishara and Weisstub (2021).

This genetic approach does not deny the complementarity of associated variables, that is, a variety of emotional inputs and environmental impacts. However, over time, and after the investment of vast sums of money in research, the hope of clearly identifying suicide risk solely based on biomarkers has waned. Research institutions and funders are now investing in the development of complex epigenetic models to potentially predict suicidal behaviours (e.g., van Heeringen and Mann, 2014), or looking at the promise of genome-wide association studies (GWAS) to scan the entire genome in large populations for variants that might be associated with a particular phenotype.

There has been no identification of a single gene or group of genes associated with suicidal ideation, suicide attempts, or deaths across multiple studies (Lutz *et al.*, 2017). Contemporary research indicates that no single gene or combination of genes can be 'responsible for suicidal ideation, suicide attempts or suicide across multiple studies ... despite a few reports confirming associations between genes identified in genome-wide studies (GWAS) ... genes of interest frequently fail to pass rigorous reproducibility and significance testing' (Turecki *et al.*, 2019, p. 4). Suicide presently falls into the category of complex conditions that may be associated with a combination of several genetic variants and environmental factors, with patterns of heritability that are uncertain and unclear.

5.1   Genetics and the Heritability of Suicide

The earliest studies of the heritability of suicide were case reports of concordant twins by Dr Benjamin Rush (1812). These findings cannot be confirmed because monozygosity and same-sex dizygosity were not identified until the 1930s. Kallmann (1953) reported a monozygotic concordance rate of 5.6% (1/18) versus a dizygotic concordance rate of 0% (0/21). Later twin studies arrived at a heritability factor of 30–50% (Fu *et al.*, 2002, Tidemalm *et al.*, 2011). However, in the countries where the studies occurred, 90% of people who had died by suicide suffered from a diagnosable mental disorder (Arsenault-Lapierre *et al.*, 2004). When the heritability of mental disorders was taken into consideration, the calculations of the heritability decreased to 17–36% (Tidemalm *et al.*, 2011).

The twin studies were complemented by evidence of family clustering. Children of parents who had died by suicide were at a higher risk, although less than 5% of people who died by suicide had a parent who died by suicide (Burrell *et al.*, 2018). Although there is a higher suicide risk in families where there was a previous death by suicide, this is not a clear indication of either a direct or an important genetic component. A great number of suicide research studies have determined that there is an imitation effect due to exposure to suicides (Crepeau-Hobson and Leech, 2014; Niedzwiedz *et al.*, 2014; Stack, 2005), which offers a nongenetic explanation for increased suicide risk in families. Moreover, it is common sense, and supported by empirical data, that the experience of the loss of a parent by suicide contributes to increased vulnerability to develop mental health problems, and difficulty in coping with traumatic events (Djelantik *et al.*, 2020; Hua *et al.*, 2019; Sveen and Walby, 2008).

There are some single-gene disorders, called 'Mendelian disorders', and there are diseases that are caused by variants of a single locus that segregate with a recognisable pattern within families. In the inception period of genetic suicidology research decades ago, vast sums of money were invested to isolate genetic 'determinants' of suicidal behaviours. However, what has developed are more complex deterministic models where genes are influenced by early-life experiences, and other characteristics are also associated with elevated suicide risk such as mental health disorders, substance abuse, and impulsivity. Researchers have turned to polygenetic and epigenetic approaches where the relative contributions of multiple genes are studied statistically, and where life experiences are considered to alter gene expression (e.g., McGowan *et al.*, 2009). Suicidologists have produced biopsychosocial models of suicide risk in which early life adversity (e.g., neglect, or physical or sexual abuse), together with genetic characteristics, result in epigenetic changes that thereafter reveal themselves in genetic expression throughout the life cycle (Turecki *et al.*, 2019). Thus, what is encoded in the genome is expressed when the person faces adversity, stress, and psychopathology. This then increases risk of suicidal behaviours.

Researchers continue attempting to 'identify and predict' based on an overlapping of genetic and epigenetic factors (Mann *et al.*, 2006). In addition to using genetic testing to help determine suicide risk, other biomarkers have been studied for their potential in predicting suicide risk and understanding the 'biological substrates' of suicidal behaviours. A recent review (Sudol and Mann, 2017) concluded that the biomarkers that appear 'promising' include indices of serotonergic function, inflammation, neuronal plasticity, and lipids.

5.2 The Promise of GWAS

For many, the lack of replicability of past genetics suicide research, and of behavioural genetics in general, will no longer be an issue as new technologies are perfected for genome-wide association studies. GWAS scan the entire genome for variants that might be associated with a particular phenotype (Hardy and Singleton, 2009; Hirschhorn and Daly, 2005). GWAS permits genotyping hundreds of thousands to over a million single nucleotide polymorphisms (SNPs) across the whole genome. Because the size of the association between individual SNPs is generally small, huge sample sizes are used to identify statistically significant associations. For example, the first GWAS study of schizophrenia, which compared 9,395 people with the diagnosis and a control group of 12,462, found 13 SNPs that appeared to differ between the cases and controls (Schizophrenia Psychiatric Genome-Wide Association Study (GWAS) Consortium, 2011). When the sample size was increased to 36,989 cases and 113,075 controls, 128 SNPs were identified (Schizophrenia Working Group of the Psychiatric Genomics Consortium, 2014). It has been estimated based on quantitative genomic restricted maximum likelihood (GREML) analyses that there are 8,300 SNPs associated with schizophrenia, which would take gigantic samples to identify (Ripke *et al.*, 2013).

5.3 Are There Intrinsic Limitations of Genetics Research to Predict Human Behavioural Traits?

Based on GWAS research findings, Chabris *et al.* (2015) concluded that behavioural phenotypes are much more polygenic than physical and medical traits – that is, they have many more genetic variants, each accounting for a much smaller share of the variability. This led them to propose a 'Fourth Law of Behaviour Genetics' to add to the widely discussed 'Three Laws of Behaviour Genetics' proposed by (Turkheimer, 2000).

Turkheimer's three laws were (2000, p. 160):

1. All human behavioural traits are heritable.
2. The effects of being raised in the same family are smaller than the effects of genes.
3. A substantial portion of the variation in complex human behavioural traits is not accounted for by the effects of genes and families.

Chabris *et al.* (2015, p. 305) provided evidence for a fourth law, based on their review of GWAS research:

4. A typical human behavioural trait is associated with very many genetic variants, each of which accounts for a very small percentage of the behavioural variability.

Thus far, attempts to calculate polygenic risk scores (PRSs) using GWAS to accurately discriminate among the behaviours of groups of people have failed. This is usually blamed on differences in environmental conditions. The European Commission's review of GWAS research concluded that PRSs have no, or only limited, predictive accuracy in samples with different ancestry or environmental background and have very limited use for individual prediction (Angers *et al.*, 2019). Considering the use of GWAS research as it could be applied to suicide, with a sufficiently large sample, it is likely that one would find a very large number of SNPs that account for such a small percentage of the behavioural variability that they would be useless for prediction.

Even if suicide as a behavioural outcome were as homogeneous as schizophrenia, which we argue is far from the case, we would need to conduct genetic analyses of at least one out of five of the 800,000 people who die by suicide in the world annually, and probably many more than that, to allow the identification of tens of thousands of SNPs, each contributing a miniscule amount to predicting suicide, with limited combined ability to discriminate between suicide and non-suicide groups and little hope of predicting individual behaviours. The costs to obtain GWAS analyses on hundreds of thousands of suicide deaths and a comparable control group would exceed the worldwide investment in suicide prevention, with no promise of useful results. Although this is the current situation, one can reflect on the ethical considerations raised by any future research developments that would permit the prediction of suicide in individuals, and the ethical considerations associated with the use of these methods.

5.4   The Assumption of Commonalities in Suicide and Implications for Prediction

Studies of genetics and suicide are often based on a presupposition that an analogy can be drawn between suicide and medical domains such as cardiology and cancer, where genetic testing has sometimes created opportunities for the prevention or treatment of life-threatening conditions. The analogy is faulty because, unlike what is true in these physical domains, there are no clearly observable chemical, electrical, anatomical, or biological indicators that provide evidence of the presence of a disease or pathology and could be used to reliably validate the efficacy of a predictive test before a death by suicide. A suicide may be identified after the person dies, but the identification is based on the nature of the person's actions that led to the death, if they had been intentionally initiated by the deceased. The nature of the injuries that caused the death does not indicate whether the death occurred by accident or suicide. Even though there are debates about the fine points concerning the level of pathology and diagnosis within medical specialties, in non-suicide medicine, disease pathology that confirms the diagnosis is clearly observable both before and after death.

Suicide is not a disease or mental illness, although it is listed as a possible symptom or outcome of several mental illness diagnoses. It is commonly accepted that many people consider suicide or 'decide' to kill themselves. However, only a very small proportion of people who consider ending their lives will attempt the act. Indeed, the most accurate verbal and written tests to predict suicide are replete with false positives (Chan *et al.*, 2016). Research on suicide risk assessment scales has found that the best predictor variables are responses to direct questions about intentions and plans to go forward with the act. Still, a meta-analysis of research found that 60% of people who attempt suicide will deny their suicidal intentions beforehand (McHugh *et al.*, 2019).

An implicit premise when one seeks genetic indicators of suicide risk is the belief that there are significant commonalities in people who die by suicide; that the phenomenon of 'suicide' can be considered as a whole, rather than as an end result of a wide variety of causal pathways and different pathological aetiologies. Shneidman (1973), one of the most influential pioneers in understanding suicide, proposed that there are common cognitions and emotions associated with suicide, such as feelings of hopelessness and suffering, accompanied by the subjective cognitive beliefs that the suffering is interminable and nothing other than death can end the emotional pain. Shneidman found that these characteristic feelings and cognitions can fluctuate greatly, even when a suicide attempt is 'decided' and imminent, or in progress. This explains how talking with a helpline counsellor can make the person feel better, envision other ways to cope with the situation, regain hope, and decide to live.

The premise that suicidal people have much in common has been challenged clinically and empirically. For example, Jean Baechler (1975), in *Les suicides* (The Suicides), describes a large variety of reasons that people die by suicide, each with its own explanations and associated pathologies. For Baechler, suicide can be an act to end suffering, to seek revenge, to punish oneself or others, to blackmail others, to cry out for help, to sacrifice oneself, and it can even be enacted as a risk-taking game. If one accepts the premise of diversity in suicidal aetiologies, suicidal people who impulsively kill themselves when risking capture for a crime, who attempt suicide after a girlfriend abandons them, who hallucinate voices during a psychotic episode, who see everything as useless during an untreated or poorly treated clinical depression, or who kill themselves while inebriated have little in common.

5.5   Possible Reasons for Genetic Testing as Related to Suicide Risk

Assuming that the theoretical and practical issues we have raised could be somehow resolved by technological advances and new theoretical insights, would testing to predict suicide risk then be useful and could its use be justified? There are a variety of motives for genetic testing. Testing that has utility in prediction can be divided into presymptomatic and predisposition testing. In presymptomatic testing, a healthy person is tested for a condition that the person is going to develop, but with a delayed onset. In predisposition testing, a positive result indicates that a person is more likely than others to develop a condition. A genetic evaluation of a person with a family history of Huntington's disease is an example of presymptomatic testing. A positive result indicates that the person will eventually develop the disease. This knowledge could be useful in influencing a person making a life decision such as having children or making choices about treatment, even though the exact timing of the disease onset is uncertain. Currently there is no way of preventing or delaying the emergence of Huntington's disease.

In contrast, predisposition genetic testing has played an important role in determining the risk of developing certain types of cancer. A positive result is often tantamount to call for increased surveillance, but by no means is it a firm indication that the cancer will occur. The test simply indicates that a person has a statistically greater risk. A negative result does not indicate that the person will not get cancer, but rather that the risk is similar to the general population, which may not be negligible (Hagenkord *et al.*, 2020; McPherson, 2006).

Genetic researchers are very hesitant to suggest that suicide exists in a presymptomatic state when undertaking a genetic profile. They contend modestly that a genetic profile can provide an indication of increased risk or predisposition for suicide to occur at a later time. The degree of certainty overall is unknown. If genetic testing is of use to predict suicide, it is for predisposition risk assessment.

5.6 Guidelines for Determining if Genetic Testing Is Ethically Acceptable in Relation to Suicide

If it ever becomes possible to use genetic testing to predict suicide, there are a large number of ethical guidelines that specify when genetic tests should be used in medicine and when they are contraindicated. Pitini *et al.* (2018) identified 29 frameworks published between 2000 and 2017 and concluded that the majority were based on the ACCE framework developed by the Centers for Disease Control Office of Public Health Genomics (2010). The acronym ACCE is based on the four main criteria for evaluating a genetic test: analytic validity; clinical validity; clinical utility; and ethical, legal, and social implications. ACCE proposes 44 specific questions that concern the nature of the disorder, the nature of the test, and clinical scenarios as well as analytic and clinical validity, clinical utility, and the associated ethical, legal, and social issues. The ACCE process applies to both Mendelian disorders and complex diseases.

In the case where a single highly predictive gene is identified, ethical considerations may preclude genetic testing. If the test has high sensitivity, specificity, and clinical validity, one should also pose questions about its clinical utility: What is the natural history of the disorder with and without intervention? What is the impact of positive test results on patient care, in terms of measurable benefits from an available intervention or treatment with concurrent consideration of ethical, legal, and social issues? What is known about stigmatisation, discrimination, privacy/confidentiality, personal, family, and social issues, in light of the presence or absence of relevant safeguards?

Assessing the usefulness of genetic tests for conditions where there are complex relationships with genetic markers is even more challenging. When the biomarkers are an actual indicator of the presence of a disease, results are where one can dichotomise diagnostic tests as being positive or negative, and subsequently determine parameters of the test's performance, such as its sensitivity, specificity, and predictive value. When we are dealing with probabilistic prognosis, as is the case with suicide, the genotype is a risk factor that indicates susceptibility to a future disease that is not currently present. In these circumstances, there is no consensus on a metric against which to determine the accuracy of the test results (Wright and Kroese, 2010).

In order to use any genetic test for prediction, one must first determine its ability to identify the genetic variance of interest accurately and reliably in a clinical laboratory. This 'analytic validity' includes assessment of sensitivity (how often there are false-negative results for the presence of genetic variance), analytic specificity (false-positive results), difference between laboratories conducting the test and 'assay robustness' (reproducibility among different people conducting the test, using different reagent lots and instruments, differences associated with ambient temperature and so on; Teutsch et al., 2009). A test that has good analytic validity must then be assessed for its clinical validity: its ability to identify and predict accurately the disorder of interest. The test must have good clinical sensitivity.

In the case of genetic testing for Huntington's disease, there is strong clinical validity. In other diagnoses, however, the clinical validity of genetic tests has been determined to be deficient – for example, testing for mutations of the BRCA1 gene, which suggests a predisposition for breast or prostate cancer. The clinical utility of a genetic test refers to the scientific evidence that testing will measurably improve the clinical outcome or add value to patient management decision-making. In some instances, even if there is not a cure or treatment, there still may be clinical utility, since the quality of life can be improved, and individuals may be able to make better life choices based on their assumed risk.

Since suicide is a behavioural outcome with no known physical precursors, it is misleading to compare the clinical utility of genetic testing for suicide with some cancers or with Huntington's disease, where genetic information can assist in improving survival, quality of life, and decision-making. Even in the case of easily diagnosable medical conditions with a strong genetic basis, genetic testing might not provide clinical utility of any consequence. For example, type 2 diabetes has a strong genetic basis; 70% of monozygotic twins who have a twin that is diabetic will become diabetic, compared with 20–30% of dizygotic twins (Lyssenko and Laakso, 2013). Over 65 genetic variants have been identified that increase the risk of type 2 diabetes by 10–30%. Several studies that combine information from all genetic risk variants for diabetes have genetic risk scores from 0.54 to 0.63, which indicates that they are very poor predictors of the risk of an individual having the disease. Furthermore, when one examines clinical risk factors such as obesity, exercise, and blood test indicators, genetics adds very little to predicting type 2 diabetes. Therefore, despite clear evidence that type 2 diabetes has a strong genetic basis, to date genetic testing has been found to be of no use in helping to predict the risk of developing this disease.

When one assesses whether it is ethical to use genetic testing or other biomarkers to assess a predisposition for suicide, the preliminary question is whether genetic tests can significantly contribute to prediction. We have argued that this is inherently impossible because of the nature of suicide and the limited ability of genes to predict human behaviours in general. In this context, it is important to note that most research on genetics and suicide has associated genetic factors with suicidal ideation or nonlethal suicide attempts. This is because death by suicide is a rare phenomenon and there are relatively few genetic data available on people who die by suicide. However, since the incidence of suicide attempts is at least 20 times higher than actual deaths by suicide, and given the fact that it is possible to screen large numbers of the population for attempts, the attempters can be studied. Finally, since there is a much larger population of people who consider suicide, it is much easier to study suicide ideators and their genetic makeup than to study people who actually die by suicide.

Current research suggests that suicidal ideation, suicide attempts, and death by suicide are not essentially a part of a continuum. The people who attempt suicide and do not die have been shown to possess a different aetiology and characteristics than people who die from suicide (DeJong *et al.*, 2010; Joo *et al.*, 2016). Research (genetic or otherwise) on suicide ideators and attempters may not help us understand or identify those people who are at risk of dying by suicide. One would expect that the genetic study of ideators, attempters, and people who die by suicide should be separate domains of genetics research.

One of the key elements in the ACCE process of determining whether to use a particular genetic test is a consideration for whether the testing is likely to result in preventive treatment. A corollary is the obligation to avoid harm. If test results reveal large numbers of false positives (low sensitivity), then many people who are not actually susceptible will believe that they are at risk. The identification of someone as being at risk of suicide may have harmful consequences. Both falsely and accurately identifying people as suicidal can lead to stigmatisation. The labelling of anyone as being suicide-prone can have a profound impact on the person's quality of life and human potential. Being identified as suicide-prone can lead to increased anxiety for individuals and their families, harmful effects of discrimination in education and employment opportunities, and social ostracisation, e.g., in marriage arrangements, business partnerships, and trusted societal positions.

A negative result from a genetic test is no guarantee or assurance that a person will not be suicidal, unless there is high specificity. However, genetic testing for complex relationships with epigenetic associations will have to have low specificity because of the diversity of other factors involved. Having a negative test result would indicate that the risk is equivalent to the risk of the general population, but offers no indication that a person will have a lower than average risk. Although this can be explained to people who receive negative results, this could create a false sense of protection. Individuals who receive negative results may not seek help, even during a suicidal crisis. Family and friends may ignore warning signs due to the 'negative' results.

Are there effective interventions to prevent suicide in people who are not at imminent risk? The challenging question is how to establish the benefits from the early identification of risk, particularly if there is no evidence of any effective intervention. When people are already actively exhibiting suicidal thoughts, tendencies, or desires, there are proven treatments: crisis intervention, psychotherapy, pharmacotherapy, and the treatment of associated risk factors, such as clinical depression and other mental health and substance abuse problems. The compelling point is that one does not need a genetic test to determine risk when there are behavioural indicators of imminent suicide or self-harm. There are no data that demonstrate the utility of adding genetic information when risk is imminent or before clear indicators of suicidal intentions are present.

Genetic research on suicide to date has focused on comparative analyses with control groups – for example, those who have died accidentally. Data on the sensitivity and specificity of using genetic information have rarely been provided. Genetic studies are conducted using post-hoc analyses of brain tissue after death. However, researchers rarely report data on the incidence of the same genetic markers in the general population. To date, there are no prospective longitudinal studies using genetic data to predict a future suicide.

Cornel *et al.* (2014) cite many examples where the burdens of using genetic testing for physical illnesses have contraindicated their use. These include situations where the financial costs of the tests were thought to outweigh potential benefits, where there were negative impacts of false reassurance after negative results, where there were feelings of doom or hopelessness when results were positive, and where there were substantial psychosocial risks of negative changes in family and social relationships upon getting genetic information. Any assessment of the usefulness of genetic testing for suicide should adhere to the ACCE guidelines and carefully evaluate the potential negative consequences of knowing the test results.

5.7 A Contemporary Challenge: Lay Use of Genetic Tests to Identify Suicide Risk

Whether or not physicians ever use genetic tests to identify suicide risk, individuals can now obtain genetic test results online and by post, without contact with the medical system. The results of home genetic testing are provided for a fee to a variety of organisations that track family ancestry, provide information on genetic risks for specific diseases, and map family trees. The number of personal DNA tests has dramatically increased in recent years (Mordor Intelligence Inc., 2020). Along with exponentially growing use, there have been controversies about which variants or mutations to test for and the validity of conclusions or predictions about the heritability of the disorders in question (Wright and Kroese, 2010). It may be that, regardless of the validity of using genetic tests to predict suicide risk and the potential dangers associated with the use of these tests, private companies will offer genetic tests for suicide risk in the uncontrolled internet environment, with the consequential risks we have outlined.

5.8 The Obligation for Clinicians to Test and to Inform Individuals and Families of Results (with or Without Consent)

In the event that genetic tests may eventually evolve to a higher predictive and reliable level of findings, will medical and mental health professionals have an obligation to convey the information? There is an extensive legal literature on the duty to inform in the event that there is a 'dangerousness' element attached, even implicitly, in the findings (Chaimowitz *et al.*, 2000). In the medical community, there is a normative tradition of presenting the outcome of tests in cases of Trisomy 21 (Down syndrome) and cases of Huntington's disease, although there has been limited legal attention to situations where specificity is low.

In 1983, the US President's Commission for the Study of Ethical Problems in Medicine, Biomedical, and Behavioural Research identified four conditions that must be met before patient's genetic information should be disclosed without consent:

1. Reasonable efforts to solicit voluntary consent to disclosure have failed.
2. There is a high probability that harm will occur if information was withheld, and the disclosed information will be used to avert harm.
3. The harm that identifiable individuals would suffer is serious.
4. Appropriate precautions are taken to ensure that only the genetic information needed is divulged.

Subsequently, the commission added an additional condition: that there is no other reasonable way to avert the harm or risk. In the event that reliable and valid genetic test information about suicide risk becomes available, disclosure of the information should meet the requirements of the President's Commission conditions or similar ethical criteria.

5.9   Specific Issues Concerning Testing Children for Risk of Suicide Later in Life

If genetic testing for suicide is proven to be beneficial, there are specific issues to consider when the tests involve children. Guidelines for predictive testing of children for an adult-onset condition indicate that testing should not be undertaken if there are no medical interventions that are useful following a positive test result. Three main reasons have been identified. First, minors are not considered capable of making an informed choice about testing. Thus, testing would constitute an infringement on their integrity and their future autonomy. Second, it can be argued that this is a prima facie breach of a minor's confidentiality. Third, there is an indisputable psychosocial impact that is more harmful to a minor once a determination is made that he or she is at risk for later onset. The impact can be dramatic and irreversible.

There is no research evidence that childhood interventions can be preventive of suicidal ideations, attempts, or an eventual death by suicide. If there is no scientifically validated anticipated benefit to minors, there is no ethical justification for conducting predictive testing. Children rarely attempt, or die from, suicide before adolescence (World Health Organization, 2021b). In the very uncommon situations where children do die by suicide, there is also a debate among professionals as to whether or not the child truly was capable of understanding the nature of the act (Miller, 2019; Mishara, 1999a). Research has demonstrated that young children are not able to conceive of their death as a final state from which there is no return (Mishara, 1999a). In older children, who do in fact understand the irreversibility of death, there is often the belief that after dying they would go on experiencing life (Mishara, 1999a).

Presymptomatic and predictive genetic testing of minors should only be performed when established and effective medical treatments can be offered: 'when testing provides scope for treatment which to an essential degree prevents, defers or alleviates the outbreak of disease or the consequences of the outbreak of disease' (Borry et al., 2006).

Even when medical professionals refrain from genetic testing of children, parents may seek direct consumer genetic testing without legal or ethical constraints through the Internet. In contrast to medical settings, where testing is usually accompanied by counselling or special education, the conveyance of results in consumer genetic testing is unregulated. The risks of misinterpretation of test results are substantial. Although genetic markers for suicide risk are not currently available to consumers, unregulated genetic suicide testing could be offered without reliability, validity, or proven benefits.

Studies have demonstrated that there is a strong interest among the general population in predictive testing of children, even in instances where there is an apparent lack of preventive interventions. In reviewing attitudes concerning genetic testing in psychiatry, Lawrence and Appelbaum (2011) stated that many people are ready to alter their lifestyles and plans for child-rearing in response to test results. These researchers express concerns about discrimination and people being potentially unable to cope with the results from their genetic profile. The authors concluded that genetic testing in psychiatry will attract a large following despite the evidence indicating significant limitations.

5.10   General Discussion and Conclusions

We have argued in this chapter that genetic testing to assess suicide risk is fraught with difficulties. There is no empirical evidence of its usefulness, and there are grave concerns for its potential negative impacts, even if genetic testing were to be proven accurate. Because of the low incidence of suicide, its multi-determined nature, and the multiple causal pathways that lead to suicide, it may be inherently impossible to identify genetic markers that will add to the predictive value of current behavioural and clinical assessments.

Suicide is more likely to occur in some families. However, this does not indicate a preponderant genetic or biological explanation. The relationship between genetics and suicide is complex; multiple genetic components, epigenetically modified by early life experiences, may increase vulnerability to suicide in a manner that we may someday be better able to accurately understand. The family-associated risk is further complicated by research showing that social imitation increases suicide risk, as does the heritability of mental disorders and traits such as impulsiveness. To date, few studies on genetics and suicide have been replicated, and, with current methodologies, research on this topic may be inherently unreliable.

Genome-wide association studies (GWAS) indicate that behavioural disorders such as schizophrenia are associated with tens of thousands of single nucleotide polymorphisms (SNPs) across the whole genome, each contributing a miniscule amount to the prediction of differences between groups. Predicting the risk of an individual requires much more specificity and sensitivity than identifying differences between groups. Furthermore, suicide is an outcome associated with multiple psychiatric disorders, with many causal pathways to a suicide outcome. Therefore, if people who died by suicide could be identified using GWAS, vast numbers of SNPs would be identified, each contributing very little. Even if there were a 'suicide trait', it would follow Turkheimer's third law of behaviour genetics: that a substantial portion of the variation in complex human behavioural traits is not accounted for by the effects of genes and families. Turkheimer believes that heredity research is concerned with populations and their variances. This contrasts with behavioural science, which is concerned with individual people and why they behave and experience the world the way they do.

Current studies compare genetic information from people who died by suicide with people who died by another means. There have been no prospective studies of living people that try to differentiate between suicide phenotypes and others, simply because no suicide phenotype has been shown to exist. If genetic research has any hope of helping to predict suicide, a first step would be to identify a phenotype of suicide-prone individuals. We concur with researchers and theorists who believe that there are many causal pathways to suicidal behaviours, making a single suicide phenotype impossible to delineate. However, if researchers were to identify a phenotype of people at greater risk of suicide, genetic research would have a better chance of helping predict risk. That phenotype would have to be identifiable before individuals are in a crisis situation, because in a crisis simple questions about intentions can validly identify people at risk.

Currently, machine learning approaches to the analysis of big data sets using AI have shown promise in the ability to predict suicide, sometimes more accurately predicting suicide risk than clinical judgements and the use of risk assessment scales (Linthicum *et al.*, 2019). It is possible that the addition of a large quantity of genetic information could increase the predictive power of AI algorithms. Including genetic data in complex machine learning analyses of massive multivariate data sets is very different from an individual receiving a genetic test result that indicates some increased suicide risk, even if the interpretation of the result included consideration of additional epigenetic childhood risk factors.

Some researchers contend that, using genetic information, more data and advances in research methodologies will lead to a deeper understanding of suicide and better prediction of suicidal behaviour. If future advances in genetics and epigenetics research were to identify valid and reliable indicators of increased suicide risk, before people had clearly identifiable behavioural indications that they were suicidal, would the use of genetic testing be ethically justified? Regardless of the predictive ability of genetic tests, the impact of false positives, even if limited, is consequential. Receiving either positive or negative results may do more harm than good. Until we have reason to believe that the benefits of genetic testing outweigh the potential harm, genetic testing should not be used to predict suicide, except in the context of research that examines group differences. It is imperative to avoid negative effects on individuals and their families.

The early debates in behavioural genetics involved heated clashes between people espousing racialised determinism and those favouring commitments to individual freedom and progressive social values. Philosophers committed to a notion of free will argue against the reduction of life-ending choices to an amalgam of environmental, genetic, and biological explanations. They may contend that suicide is a prerogative and right that must be respected. Predicting any serious human action challenges conceptions of free will, particularly when it involves life-or-death choices.

Regardless of empirical and ethical concerns, genetic testing provided by private companies directly to consumers is increasing exponentially. Unregulated commercial genetic test companies could offer suicide risk assessments. Service providers include disclaimers about the limits of the tests and caution about their interpretation. Nevertheless, common sense suggests that consumers who receive suicide test results outside medical settings will be at much greater risk of misinterpreting them. Misunderstanding the limitations of genetic findings could lead to increased anxieties and unfounded apprehensions, which could precipitate unnecessary and unwise life-changing choices. Consumer-protection legislation should consider laws and guidelines for using genetic information to predict suicide risk.

We conclude that it is unlikely that genetic testing will be able to reliably help identify people at risk of suicide. This is because of the inherent limitations of current behavioural genetics research and the fact that suicide is a behaviour, not a phenotype, and that it can result from many different causal pathways. If we imagine a future possibility of increasing the accuracy of genetic or epigenetic suicide prediction, ethical imperatives remain. We must refrain from using screening in the absence of effective preventive treatments. We also need to avoid the potential harm from accurately or inaccurately identifying people as suicide-prone, since this information can have an emotional impact, influence important decisions people make, and affect how they are treated by others.

6

• • • • • •

Suicide and Civil Commitment

Throughout the Western world, extensive involuntary commitment of the mentally ill has been statutory or customary practice for centuries. Despite massive deinstitutionalisation in the second half of the twentieth century and decriminalisation of suicide attempts in most jurisdictions, people considered a danger to themselves or others can still be hospitalised against their will worldwide (see Chapter 7). This chapter, expanding upon Mishara and Weisstub (2022), traces the changing criteria for forced institutionalisation and treatment in the context where countries are legalising medically assisted death for people who suffer only from a mental disorder. We analyse the conflicting values and premises that pit benevolent concerns for the protection of vulnerable people against trends towards blanket recognition of autonomous decision-making in all spheres of life.

6.1 The Transition from Paternalistic Mass Incarceration, to Limiting Forced Hospitalisation, to Considering 'Dangerousness'

In the early modern era following rapid industrialisation, the problem of managing those who did not fit in, including those who were mentally challenged due to birth, trauma, or diagnosable illnesses, resulted in the creation of institutions where a substantial population was incarcerated, sometimes indefinitely. Only in the mid-1960s did we observe a rapid transformation away from the warehousing of the mentally infirm. Deinstitutionalisation began in northern Italy in 1961, where Professor Franco Basaglia, a charismatic leader in psychiatry, organised the Movement for Democratic Psychiatry (Foot, 2015; Goodwin, 1997). After numerous community support experiments in Arezzo, Ferrara, Gorizia, Perugia Trieste, Verona and other cities principally in Northern Italy between 1961 and 1978, the reforms culminated in the *Legge Basaglia* (Basaglia Law, 1978), which contained directives for closing all psychiatric hospitals and their replacement by a range of community services (Istituzione del Servizio Sanitario Nazionale, 1978). During the same period, other Western European countries initiated similar reforms. In the United States (USA), there were numerous exposés of painfully inadequate and dehumanising conditions. Sociologists wrote about discriminatory practices at many institutions, showing that public prejudice against mental illness was derogatory and demeaning (Dyck, 2011; Gijswijt-Hofstra, 2005).

Since the 1960s, pharmaceutical advances and policy changes in Western countries have generally replaced confinement in large mental hospitals with referral to community services, although those community services are often underfunded. The depopulation of asylums in Italy and elsewhere led to intense political discussion and backlash (Barham, 1997; Burns, 2019; Burns and Foot, 2020; Foot, 2015). Families and communities struggled with patients' reintegration, the dilemmas of mentally ill populations who refused or did not respond to treatment, and inadequacies in community services.

When is involuntary treatment of the mentally ill ethical? In North America, the criterion of 'dangerousness' to oneself or others became the dominant basis for incarceration. Laws restricted the number of days people could be held for psychiatric assessments. There was a worldwide evolution towards accepting 'dangerousness' as the morally justified condition for removing individuals from society (Arboleda-Flórez and Weisstub, 2008).

6.2   Defining 'Dangerousness'

In the 1980s, the American Psychiatric Association articulated the basis for legislation permitting involuntary hospitalisation that emphasised the criterion of dangerousness (Appelbaum, 1994; Borecky et al., 2019; Stone and Stromberg, 1976; Stromberg and Stone, 1983; Werth, 2001). The revisions of the Mental Health Act in Canada and throughout the Commonwealth paralleled the changes in the USA. Criteria for involuntary institutionalisation included diminished capacity, a diagnosable mental disorder, and a treatable condition (Olsen, 1998). In practice, however, the emphasis was on the likelihood of harming oneself or others. The standard of dangerousness has become the key factor in civil commitment statutes throughout the USA and the Commonwealth (Coleman, 2021; Fistein et al., 2009).

Parallel to those legislative changes, psychiatrists and physicians responsible for making commitment decisions adopted defensive practices against potential malpractice suits (Groth and Boccio, 2019; Halleck, 2012; Jobes and Berman, 1993). This led to an increase in precautionary involuntary confinements of community residents, usually for a very restricted period (Kisely and Campbell, 2015; Swanson et al., 2017; Wettstein, 2003).

In Canada, the relevant statutes, which vary in nuance by province, include protections to comply with the Canadian Charter of Rights and Freedoms. The commitment process is now almost entirely in the hands of physicians, except for a few exceptions such as in Quebec, where a judicial confirmation is required. There are some variations where the committal criteria include substantial physical or mental deterioration, lack of capacity, the role of substitute decision-makers, and a prior history of mental health treatments (Gray *et al.*, 2010; O'Reilly and Gray, 2014; Perlin *et al.*, 2017).

The most recent development has been the implementation of outpatient civil commitment or court-directed mental health treatments coupled with monitoring arrangements (Segal *et al.*, 2017; Torrey and Zdanowicz, 2001). These were developed to temper the human and financial costs associated with inpatient interventions while retaining forms of legal control (Appelbaum, 2001; Segal *et al.*, 2017). The effectiveness of these alternatives has yet to be confirmed.

Legislation and judicial decisions concerning involuntary hospitalisation often refer to the International Covenant on Civil and Political Rights, enacted 16 December 1966 (UN General Assembly, 1966). This covenant provides protection against discrimination based upon physical or mental limitations and offers protections against coercive measures. Judicial decisions have also been associated with the United Nations Convention on the Rights of Persons with Disabilities (CRPD), enacted 13 December 2006 (Bartlett, 2003; MacSherry, 2010; Minkowitz, 2006; Ruissen *et al.*, 2012). The CRPD, the first human rights convention open for signature by regional organisations, affirms that persons with a wide range of disabilities must enjoy all human rights and fundamental freedoms (Bach and Kerzner, 2010).

6.3   Critiques of the Criterion of Dangerousness and the Focus on Competency

The adoption of dangerousness to oneself or others as the sole criterion for institutionalisation has drawn critiques (Bartlett, 2003; Crowe and Carlyle, 2003; Maris, 1992; Saya *et al.*, 2019). Research has indicated that the prediction of dangerousness was unreliable (Mulder *et al.*, 2016). Therefore, individuals were seen to be held against their will without proper scientific rationale (Ho, 2014). As a result, in recent decades, *competency* has become the guiding component for involuntary commitment and enforced treatment.

Competency can fluctuate over time, even within a matter of minutes or hours. Competency can change with transient or chronic stressors, with physical pain, with medical conditions, and with the ingestion of psychoactive substances. Blanket determinations of incompetency are currently increasingly rare. Competency assessment, now detailed in most mental health acts, involves measuring capacity in specific areas such as financial matters and medical treatments. There is no single common-law test for general mental or decision-making competency. Medical competency assessors have reached high levels of inter-rater reliability, even with regard to psychiatric treatment decisions (Dawson and Szmukler, 2006; Ruissen *et al.*, 2012). Regardless, society is challenged by patients who resist treatment who are not actively or acutely dangerous to themselves or others, but lack the resources (housing, employment, social support) for a viable life in the community.

There have been a number of academic proposals to abolish all forms of involuntary commitment and to restrict incarceration to clearly articulated instances of competency failure (Brito and Ventura, 2019; Buchanan, 2004; Cairns *et al.*, 2005; Dawson and Szmukler, 2006; Szmukler and Holloway, 1998). Would such a solution be practical and just? Where there is a threat of harm to others, the criminal process would be an obvious alternative. However, this could result in the criminalising of a certain sector of the mentally ill population. It is argued by defenders of the competency test that criteria for the determination of competency are far more precise and well researched than the more amorphous criteria of dangerousness, which have been found to lack reliability in numerous studies (Carpiniello *et al.*, 2020; Dawson and Szmukler, 2006).

The use of involuntary commitment or incompetency determinations will never be uniform, regardless of the criteria, since clinical practices inevitably involve subjective judgements. Within the mental health profession, paternalism is still intrinsic to everyday practices. Clinicians are confronted with ambiguous criteria and highly emotional demands from patients, families, and community organisations. Decisions about involuntary confinement always occur in the context of interpersonal relationships. Abstract rules for involuntary commitment will never achieve a credible level of application or integration, independent of the relationships that exist between healers and patients. Some have described this as the challenge of relational approaches in contrast to rights-based ethical models (Nicolini *et al.*, 2018; Olsen, 2003).

6.4 Extrajudicial Practices When There Is Danger to Self: The Case of Helplines

Outside the judicial realm, when the life of an individual is in danger, interventions against a person's will to preserve life can vary, dependent upon the ethical premises of the helpers (Mishara and Weisstub, 2005). We have, in Chapter 2, contrasted the life-saving practices of suicide prevention helplines in the USA and the United Kingdom (UK) (Mishara and Weisstub, 2010). The US helplines have an active rescue policy, obliging centres to trace and localise calls from people at imminent risk of attempting suicide and sending police and ambulances, even when the callers state they do not want assistance. This has been justified ethically by the social responsibility to save lives, as well as by the argument that those rescued were subsequently grateful for the intervention.

The UK Samaritans' helpline policy, which we described in Chapter 2, insists that they do everything possible to convince the caller to accept rescue. However, their policy is to respect the caller's desires, based upon the ethical premise that it is for the caller to make the ultimate decision. In addition, the Samaritans reason that if they did not respect callers' confidentiality, other suicidal callers would be dissuaded from using their life-saving services.

In 2020, the US National Suicide Prevention Lifeline network changed its policies, and they now limit sending help against a person's will to the most extreme situations. Some branches of Samaritans in the UK have moved towards the occasional acceptance of sending help when callers have initiated a potentially lethal attempt, and where their mental state is compromised, thus invoking perceived incompetency as a justification for intervention. The aforementioned policies highlight that ethical premises influence suicide-prevention practises. The extent to which autonomy in decision-making is respected can determine what, when, and how help may be provided, with or without considering competency.

6.5   Force-Feeding at Guantánamo Bay

Life-threatening situations occur in carceral institutions in many author-itarian countries where there is torture. In some instances, death results from hunger strikes and the lack of life-saving interventions. The previ-ous examples in this chapter concerned people who voluntarily called a helpline. Another example concerns a similarly perilous situation, one in which the person in danger is incarcerated and is not in a voluntary inter-action with help-givers. In April 2013, a *New York Times* report described force-feeding of prisoners at the detention camp at the US naval base in Guantánamo Bay, Cuba (Lewis, 2005). The prisoners had been held for years in what were described as 'inhumane' conditions. They staged a hunger strike, stating they would 'rather die' than be incarcerated with no recourse to a judicial process. When their physical state gravely deterio-rated, the prisoners were involuntarily force-fed by the prison authorities. A flurry of articles and letters to the *New York Times* presented views on whether or not force-feeding could be justified.

Mishara (2013) presented the opinion that in suicide prevention, inter-ventions to save a life, including intrusive interventions such as pumping someone's stomach when they have ingested poison or the force-feeding of a person who has stopped eating, can be justified as a temporary meas-ure. The intrusive intervention is considered to be warranted to allow the person to survive during a crisis in order to subsequently obtain necessary treatment. In fact, only a small portion (about 10–16%) of people who are treated in hospital following a suicide attempt will make another attempt within the year after their discharge (Carroll *et al.*, 2014; Carter *et al.*, 2017; Owens *et al.*, 2002). At Guantánamo, the circumstances that motivated the hunger strike seemed unlikely to change. The US government gave no indication that the prisoners would be tried for their crimes in the foreseeable future, nor would they be permitted legal process to contest their indefinite detention without conviction.

Viewing a potentially lethal hunger strike as a political action without suicidal intent parallels analyses of the motivations of suicide bombers, who kill others for political reasons (Townsend, 2007). They anticipate their death. However, unlike individuals with suicidal intent, their goal is to kill others, using a method in which their death is an unavoidable consequence. According to interview studies of suicide bombers caught before exploding their bombs (Hassan, 2001; Post *et al.*, 2003), they simply wished to effect social change. Several authors reported that some volunteers were refused as suicide bombers because their mental health problems could lead to their discovery before the bombing (Fotion *et al.*, 2007; Scott, 2011). In the earlier example of suicide attempters calling a helpline, the question of competency may be invoked. However, the competency of the Guantánamo prisoners was not invoked. Should there be a presumption of incompetency after many years of incarceration?

6.6   Protection of Vulnerable People and the Right to Choose Death over Suffering: Medical Assistance in Dying (MAiD)

Involuntary treatment and competency concerning treatment decisions have recently become the focus in debates on expanding medical assistance in dying – euthanasia and assisted suicide – to include people whose sole reason for requesting to die is their suffering from a mental disorder.

There is concern that when mental illness is the reason for MAiD, presumed competency is being determined based on a low standard (Calati *et al.*, 2021; Okai *et al.*, 2007). Regardless of the standard for competency, there is a long-standing practice of protecting suicidal persons by hospitalisation when they are at risk of self-harm. Receiving involuntary treatment following a suicide attempt highlights the dialectic between empowering people with a mental illness to make major life decisions, and considering ethical concerns to protect vulnerable people from making decisions that have dire consequences. The following example highlights these concerns:

> In 2019, Alan Nichols, who had a history of depression, was brought by the Royal Canadian Mounted Police (RCMP) to a hospital in British Columbia; he was suffering from malnutrition and dehydration (Favaro *et al.*, 2019). His brother was informed that Alan was admitted to hospital for his own health and safety, and thereafter flew to join him. Alan told his brother to return home, which he did. A week later, a doctor informed his brother that Alan was scheduled for MAiD in eight days. The family reacted with shock and said that Alan had no serious medical condition, and that he became suicidal whenever his depression was untreated. When the family visited Alan, they stated that he was delusional and very agitated, which they attributed to ceasing to take antidepressant and anti-seizure medications. The family tried to postpone his death and begin treatment. The doctor decided that only his patient could stop the procedure. Alan Nichols died by lethal injection on 26 July 2019, with family present.

This case raises a number of legal, practical, and ethical issues. It occurred before application of the Superior Court's decision in *Truchon* (*Truchon v. Attorney General of Canada and Attorney General of Québec*, 2019), which eliminated the requirement that death be 'foreseeable' in order to have access to MAiD. One could debate whether Alan Nichols met the 2019 requirements for MAiD that death be foreseeable. According to his family, death was not imminent.

The other legal requirement for MAiD was competency. Alan Nichols was diagnosed with clinical depression. When he made the request for MAiD, he had stopped taking his medications. In Canada, a person is considered competent unless there is a legal determination to the contrary. Canadians have a legally protected right to refuse treatment. The only exception is where their life or the lives of others are in peril. No request for a judicial review of Alan Nichols' competency was made.

Although there is currently no legal obligation to do so, is there a moral obligation to consult the family when a person has chosen to die by MAiD? The doctors who approved MAiD for Alan Nichols had known him for only a few weeks. However, the family had a very different understanding of the nature of his medical history and his suicidal intentions, specifically pertaining to the relationship between refusal of medical treatments and the desire to die.

6.7   Arguments for MAiD for People with Mental Disorders

Advocates in Canada in favour of MAiD for persons for whom a mental disorder is the sole underlying medical condition (MD-SUMC) have been spearheaded by Jocelyn Downey at Dalhousie University, who convened a group of eight like-minded colleagues to make recommendations to the Canadian government in regard to MAiD for persons with MD-SUMC. Their report (The Halifax Group, 2020) proclaims that the suffering of persons with MD-SUMC can be as intense as the suffering from a terminal medical illness; therefore, those people should not be forced to endure it.

We do not contest that suffering from a mental illness may feel as intense as suffering from a physical illness. Key issues are whether interminable suffering from a mental illness is inevitable, and whether it is possible for skilled mental health professionals to determine when the prospect for recovery is hopeless. The Halifax Group (2020) recommended that persons with MD-SUMC not be excluded in amendments to the Canadian federal and Quebec MAiD legislation, since they said that excluding people with MD-SUMC from accessing MAiD is 'discriminatory on the basis of diagnosis rather than on the basis of real capacities (decisional capacity, ability to form well-considered judgments, etc.)', and that it reinforces a stigmatising view that all persons with a mental disorder need to be protected from themselves.

The Halifax Group said that people deserve relief when they experience intolerable suffering. They recommended that legislation should not add an eligibility criterion of 'unambivalent decision' to the legislation since 'there is nothing unique to MD-SUMC that would justify adding an eligibility criterion of unambivalent decision for MAiD MD-SUMC'. They only proposed adding one additional eligibility criterion for persons with MAiD MD-SUMC: that MAiD be 'well considered', to ensure that the decision to die is not impulsive. Furthermore, they recommended that provincial and territorial regulators should establish explicit standards for physicians and nurse practitioners to assess the criterion of having a grievous and irremediable medical condition and should discuss the reasons for requesting MAiD in detail. They also added that training should be provided to improve the skills of MAiD assessors and providers.

Downey and the Halifax Group deny that a mental illness is different from a physical illness and characterise beliefs that there are important differences as leading to discrimination. However, in contrast to physical illnesses, mental illnesses cannot currently be diagnosed by physiological indicators. Diagnoses are determined by talking with the patient about symptoms, and disagreements among psychiatrists over the 'true' diagnosis and prognosis are rampant. Furthermore, research clearly indicates that professionals are unable to predict the course of mental illnesses over time, whether treated or untreated.

According to research, 50–60% of people with depression or anxiety will recover without any treatment (Chin et al., 2015; Sareen et al., 2013; Whiteford et al., 2013) and 25% of people with substance abuse disorders will have unassisted recovery (Klingemann *et al.*, 2010). Even the most severe mental illnesses, such as schizophrenia, have increases and decreases in symptoms that are unpredictable. A review by Bellack (2006) concluded that 50% of people with schizophrenia meet objective criteria for recovery for significant periods during their lives, and these periods increase in frequency and duration after middle age.

If it were possible to distinguish the very few persons with a mental illness who are destined to suffer interminably from those whose suffering is treatable, it could be considered to be inhumane to deny MAiD. However, as we have discussed in previous chapters, research reveals that psychiatric professionals are incapable of accurately predicting the future course of a mental illness (The Halifax Group, 2020). Therefore, we must ask how many people we can allow to die needlessly because of inaccuracies in prognostic judgements.

In the Netherlands and Belgium (Cohen-Almagor, 2015), people with a mental disorder as the sole underlying illness may request euthanasia or assisted suicide to end their suffering. Those countries require that there be no alternative treatment available to relieve the suffering. If the physicians believe that untried treatments exist, they are obliged to deny access to MAiD. If the person then utilises the treatment and it is ineffective, the request for MAiD can be revisited. Because of these precautions, a very small proportion of people are granted a request for MAiD when the suffering is from a mental disorder. For example, in the Netherlands, in the 2015–2016 fiscal year, of the 1,100–1,150 requests for MAiD, only 60–70 were granted (Evenblij *et al.*, 2019). Most of the refusals were due to the belief that there were untried treatments available.

A suicidal person's ambivalence surrounding suicide is a justification for interventions against their will. Downey and colleagues explicitly recommend against requiring that there be little or no ambivalence in a request for MAiD. As we discussed in Chapter 1 of this book, a primary characteristic of suicides, even the most seemingly determined, is the presence of ambivalence. People may very much want to die at one moment and several hours, days, or weeks later may wish to continue living. Even during periods where a person seems convinced that death is the only option, some ambivalence is always present, and the desire to live can be strengthened.

The Halifax Group has stated that the decision needs only be 'well-considered' and that ambivalence is irrelevant. Their position assumes that because of the 'hopeless' prognosis of the mental illness, the patient would understandably have no desire to continue living with undignified mental decline (The Halifax Group, 2020). This reasoning conflates having a hopeless medical prognosis with *feeling* hopeless. Research on the reasons for choosing MAiD indicates that it is rarely due to physical suffering (Ferrand *et al.*, 2012; Nicolini *et al.*, 2018; Nuhn *et al.*, 2018; Rietjens *et al.*, 2009). Ferrand *et al.* (2012) found that 79% of patients in 789 palliative care facilities did not mention a physical symptom as the salient reason for the request for MAiD. Rather, the reason was the fear of future suffering, humiliation, and loss of control and dignity (Hendry *et al.*, 2013); for people suffering from a mental illness who requested MAiD, feeling hopeless was the primary characteristic.

In the case of physical illness, people frequently request MAiD because of anticipated suffering. This has been validated in the US states that have legalised assisted suicide. In those states, after determination by two physicians that the person's suffering is irreversible and intolerable, a person may be prescribed lethal medications. Relatively few people request assisted suicide in the USA, and requests that are made are almost exclusively related to cancer. In Oregon, where approximately 37,000 people die each year, only 290 were granted assisted suicide in 2020 (Public Health Division and Center for Health Statistics, 2020). Of the 2,518 people in Oregon who had convinced two physicians that they could not tolerate living with their suffering and had received lethal prescriptions since the law permitting assisted suicide was passed in 1998, one third (34%) never used the medication. They kept it 'in case' but died of natural causes. This confirms the omnipresence of ambivalence about dying by MAiD that is expressed by seemingly hopeless persons approved for assisted suicide, who changed their mind and had a natural death.

Proponents contend that if people with a disability are not allowed access to MAiD, 'this could be seen as stigmatizing suggesting that they lack the capacity of self-determination' (The Halifax Group, 2020, p. 20). This view contrasts with the United Nations Human Rights Office of the High Commissioner announcement made on 25 January 2021 that UN human rights experts have expressed alarm at a growing trend towards enacting legislation enabling access to medical assistance in dying, based largely on having a disability or disabling conditions:

> Under no circumstance should the law provide that it could be a well-reasoned decision for a person with a disabling condition who is not dying to terminate their life with the support of the State. ... Such legislative provisions would institutionalize and legally authorize 'ableism,' and directly violate Article 10 of the UN Convention on the Rights of Persons with Disabilities, which requires States to ensure that persons with disabilities can effectively enjoy their inherent right to life on an equal basis with others. (Forcignanò, 2021, third paragraph)

6.8 Conclusions

We can foresee heart-wrenching cases that will accentuate the moral dilemmas facing mental health professionals (Emanuel *et al.*, 2016; Kallmann, 1953; Kamisar, 1998; Lillehammer, 2002). Professionals are being confronted by patients, their families, and intimates who have divergent opinions about the legality or moral requirements presented by the simultaneous demands put before them (Thomasma and Weisstub, 2004).

In Canada the governing legal decision on competency is found in the Starson case (*Starson v. Swayze*), decided by the Supreme Court of Canada in 2003 (Sklar, 2011; Weisstub, 1990). The Court determined that a competent patient has the absolute entitlement to make what appear to be irrational decisions from the point of view of the standard of reasonableness. Entitlement is determined by a competency assessment made by mental health professionals according to an adequate standard of their profession. An equivalent rule has been adopted across the industrialised nations (Carpiniello *et al.*, 2020; Gray *et al.*, 2010).

A clear and simple statement or a precise set of criteria that lead to universally agreed determinations of competency does not exist. Families may be more familiar with the patients than physicians, who see them for a brief period. On the other hand, families may have ulterior interests (Mormont and Weissstub, 2020), manifestations of unresolved relationships, selfish financial expectations, unfounded beliefs about mental health, and, above all, different opinions about what is an acceptable amount of time when the patient is lucid, among irrational episodes. Moreover, there are differences in what is considered to constitute a patient's 'clear appreciation' with regard to the options available. All these factors are predictably cast into play in a disturbing bundle of contradictory and emotionally charged factors that may influence decision-making (Jones-Bonofiglio, 2020).

The decision to end a life at the hands of a medical professional is not the same as a decision taken by a person exercising suicide in an 'autonomous' fashion. In our contemporary society, physicians are often not familiar with the patient's medical charts and social-emotional history stretching over a lifetime. They are forced into making a decision in an ahistorical present. Practitioners are obligated to apply a law where the clinical knowledge is neither deep nor related to the person's life history, with the moral responsibility that accompanies their facilitating a lethal outcome.

Much has occurred since the latter part of the twentieth century to promote autonomy as the highest principle of the medical practitioner–patient relationship. The icon of autonomy, despite its philosophical clarity, has the associated shortcomings of moral ambiguity and conflictual values concerning fundamental beliefs about life and death (Beauchamp and Childress, 2009; Dworkin, 1986; Dworkin, 1988). The exceptions to the autonomy principle emanate from instances where a persuasive argument can be made that there are reasons to infringe upon autonomy due to a patient's apparent deficit, attributable to personal limitations, such as mental instability or addiction. John Stuart Mill, the grandfather of individual liberty, commonsensically allowed for such situations, bearing in mind that overstatement of the principle (exceptions to the rule) may be abusive of rightfully defended liberty (Allen, 2013; Donnelly, 2010; McSherry, 2012). In situations where the celebration of autonomy as a primary moral or humanistic value appears empty since it leads to ending life, a responsible society should consider the relevance of short-term interventions which may establish credible autonomy (Miller *et al.*, 2018; Weisstub and Pintos, 2008).

It may be that in a minority of situations there is rationality in the desire to die (Caplan, 2006; Hartog *et al.*, 2020; Mayo, 1986; Savulescu, 1994): for avoidance of suffering, where there are repeated lapses in the hope for a decent quality of life. However, when we speak of 'rational' suicide and the desire to die, we usually mean that the desire to die appears in that context to be understandable to others, rather than 'rational' referring to any logical or reasoned decision-making process.

Fundamental questions remain: On which side should we encourage the possibility of the likelihood of error? Is there an inherent obligation to err on the side of maintaining life (Mishara and Weisstub, 2018)? One thing is certain. There must be a process of review that allows for at least an attempt towards neutrality, to engage the inner and outer battles among patients and their healers, medical personnel, the judicial system, the next of kin, and others.

7

• • • • • • •

The Legal Status
of Suicide

At the beginning of the nineteenth century, most countries had laws that provided for punishment, including jail sentences, for people who attempted suicide. However, since the 1970s the situation has changed significantly. Not all countries have decriminalised suicide, but most, including those without punishments for attempting suicide, have laws making it a criminal offence to incite or assist a person to engage in suicidal behaviours. Mishara and Weisstub (2016) summarised the laws criminalising suicide and identified countries where attempting suicide is a punishable crime, and where aiding and abetting suicide is illegal. This chapter provides an updated overview of the worldwide legal status of suicide and suicidal behaviours as of January 2023, discusses why suicidal behaviours are punished, and presents arguments for decriminalisation of suicide.

7.1   Punishment for Attempted Suicide

Of 193 independent countries and states, 18 currently have specific laws and punishments for attempted suicide (see Table 7.1). An additional 20 countries follow Islamic or sharia law; in these countries suicide attempters may be punished although there is no specific statute. Penalties

Table 7.1. Legal status of suicide attempters in countries where penal code specifies suicide as illegal, as of 1 March 2023

COUNTRY	LEGAL SYSTEM	LEGAL DOCUMENT	SENTENCE
Bahamas	Common Law	Penal Code	**Art. 294 – Attempt to commit suicide** Where suicide is attempted: imprisonment for life.
Bangladesh	Common Law, Islamic Law	Penal Code 1860	**Art. 309 – Attempt to commit suicide** Where suicide is attempted: simple imprisonment for one or more years, or penalty of a fine, or both.
Brunei Darussalam	Islamic Law, Common Law, Traditional Law	Penal Code (Cap. 22 of 1951)	**Art. 309 – Attempt to commit suicide** Where suicide is attempted: simple imprisonment for one or more years, or penalty of a fine, or both.
Gambia	Common Law, Traditional Law	Criminal Code	**Chapter XXI.** Where suicide is attempted: the offender is guilty of a misdemeanour.
Kenya	Common Law, Islamic Law, Traditional Law	Penal Code, Ch. 63	**CH.63 S.226. Attempt to commit suicide** Where suicide is attempted: the offender is guilty of a misdemeanour.
Lebanon	Civil Law, Traditional Law	Penal Code of 1943	Imprisonment for attempted suicide.
Malawi	Common Law, Traditional Law	Penal Code, Ch. 7:01	**Art. 229 – Attempting suicide** Where suicide is attempted: the offender is guilty of a misdemeanour.

Table 7.1. (Cont.)

COUNTRY	LEGAL SYSTEM	LEGAL DOCUMENT	SENTENCE
Nigeria	Common Law, Islamic Law, Traditional Law	Northern States: Penal Code, Sharia Federal Capital Territory: Penal Code	**Act. No 25 (1960)** Where suicide is attempted: the offender is guilty of a misdemeanour, and is liable to imprisonment for 1 year. **Section 231** Where suicide is attempted: the offender is guilty of a misdemeanour, and is liable to imprisonment for 1 year.
Papua New Guinea	Traditional Law, Common Law	Criminal Code Act 1974	**Art. 311 – Attempt to commit suicide** Where suicide is attempted: the offender is guilty of a misdemeanour, and is liable to imprisonment for 1 year.
Qatar	Islamic Law, Civil Law, Common Law, Traditional Law	Penal Code, Law no. 11 of 2004.	**Art. 304 – Attempt to commit suicide** Where suicide is committed by using, executing any actions that usually lead to death: imprisonment for up to 6 months and penalty of a fine of up to 3000 riyals, or one of these two penalties.
Saint Lucia	Civil Law, Common Law	Criminal Code, no. 9 of 2004	**Art. 94 – Suicide: aiding and abetting of suicide, attempt to commit suicide** Where suicide is attempted: imprisonment for 2 years.

Table 7.1. (Cont.)

COUNTRY	LEGAL SYSTEM	LEGAL DOCUMENT	SENTENCE
Somalia	Islamic Law, Common Law	Penal Code, Decree no. 5/1962	**Art. 437 – Attempt to commit suicide** Imprisonment.
South Sudan	Common Law	Penal Code Act, 2008	**Art. 215 – Attempt to commit suicide** Where suicide is attempted: the offender is guilty of a misdemeanour, and is liable to imprisonment for 1 year.
Sudan	Islamic Law, Common Law	Penal Code, 2003	**Section 261 – Attempt to commit suicide** Where suicide is attempted: the offender is guilty of a misdemeanour, and is liable to imprisonment for 1 year.
Tonga	Common Law	Criminal Offences Act (Chap. 18)	**Art. 100 – Suicide** Where suicide is attempted: imprisonment up to 3 years.
Uganda	Common Law, Traditional Law		**Art. 210 – Attempt to commit suicide** Where suicide is attempted: the offender is guilty of a misdemeanour.
United Republic of Tanzania	Common Law, Traditional Law	Penal Code, Cap 16, 1945 (last amended 1963)	**Art. 217 – Attempt to commit suicide** Where suicide is attempted: the offender is guilty of a misdemeanour.

stipulated in the laws range from a small fine or short imprisonment to a lifelong sentence. In the seven years following the publication of the overview by Mishara and Weisstub (2016), countries repealed laws criminalising suicide (Ghana, Guyana, India, Malaysia, Pakistan, Singapore, and Sri Lanka), and suicide was decriminalised in Cyprus, an overseas territory of the United Kingdom (UK). In Table 7.1, we have not included India in the list of countries with specific laws in which there are criminal penalties for suicidal behaviours, even though those laws are still technically in force. The Indian government had originally said they would repeal the laws, but hesitated to do so. Instead, in 2017, they passed the Mental Health Care Act, in which Article 115 (1) states: 'Notwithstanding section 309 of the Penal Code, any person who attempts to commit suicide shall be presumed, unless proven otherwise, to have severe stress and shall not be tried and punished under the said Code.' Article 115 (2) continues: 'The appropriate government shall have a duty to provide care, treatment and rehabilitation to a person having severe stress and who attempted to commit suicide, to reduce the risk of recurrence of attempt to commit suicide' (The Ministry of Law and Justice, 2017, p. 77).

There is public discussion of potential upcoming legislative proposals to decriminalise suicide as this book is being written in 2023. The International Association for Suicide Prevention and the World Health Organization are actively encouraging all countries to repeal laws and traditional practices of punishing people for attempting suicide. The majority of the countries, despite having laws stipulating punishments for suicide attempts, do not prosecute or punish attempters. The situation remains complex, and practices and jurisprudence are sometimes inconsistent.

7.2   Punishment for Abetting, Aiding, or Encouraging Suicide

Most countries, including those where suicide attempts have been decriminalised, have laws making it illegal to abet, aid, or encourage suicide, but the nature of the actions that are illegal varies greatly, as does the nature of the punishments. Of the 193 countries, 142 have laws that stipulate punishments, including jail sentences, for assisting or encouraging a suicide (Mishara and Weisstub, 2016). The wording of what is covered by these laws varies greatly, and the extent of enforcement is inconsistent. Some examples of the variety of descriptions of what is illegal may be seen in a sampling of the specific wording of the laws: 'complicity in suicide' in Bhutan and several other countries; 'suicide pacts' in Kenya; 'direct provoking of a minor to suicide' in Djibouti; 'driving someone to suicide or make a suicide attempt by way of threatening, cruel treatment or systematic humiliation of human dignity for the victim' in Kazakhstan, Tajikistan, Ukraine, Uzbekistan, and Kyrgyzstan; '[to] force, seduce, maintain or induce children or youth to commit suicide' in Taiwan; 'causing someone to commit suicide' in Armenia; 'any person who cruelly treats, constantly intimidates, ill-treats and humiliates a person dependent on him/her, inducing the latter to commit suicide' in Vietnam; 'aids or instigates a child or person who is unable to understand the nature of his act or who is unable to control his act, to commit suicide' in Thailand.

7.3 Impact of Decriminalisation of Attempted Suicide

There are no data or case reports indicating that decriminalisation increases suicides; in fact, suicide rates tend to decline in countries after decriminalisation. However, it may occur that decriminalisation will result in increased reporting of suicides once the fear of legal recriminations for attempting suicide is eliminated. In some countries, the political realities are such that decriminalisation is unlikely to take place, despite recognition by many that suicide should be treated as a mental health problem rather than as a criminal behaviour. For example, in Lebanon, both the Moslem and Christian political parties have not found it politically acceptable to change the laws about suicide, but these laws are rarely enforced.

Even in countries where suicide has been decriminalised, there are cases where people have been jailed for attempting suicide. In the United States

(USA) in 2011, Bei Bei Shuai was arrested and prosecuted for murder after she attempted suicide while pregnant; the child died shortly after birth (Pilkington, 2011). She faced sentences of up to 20 years in jail or the death penalty. She was freed in 2013 following a massive media campaign, after agreeing to plead guilty to criminal recklessness. People who attempt suicide by a car 'collision' may be prosecuted for voluntary manslaughter if an occupant of the other car or a bystander dies in the crash. In collision suicides, voluntary manslaughter can be invoked. For example, in England under Section 2 of the Homicide Act (Government of the United Kingdom, 1957) when one uses the defence of diminished responsibility in order to claim that the death was manslaughter rather than intentional homicide, the defendant must have suffered from an 'abnormality of mind' at the time of the killing, in the process of attempting suicide. These situations indicate that even if suicide attempts are decriminalised, there is always the risk of prosecution for provoking or causing harm, either intentional or unintentional, to others as a secondary consequence of a suicide attempt.

In some instances, military personnel who attempt suicide may be prosecuted in military courts. In the USA, Private Lazzaric Caldwell (Dishneau, 2015), who, according to court records, suffered from depression and post-traumatic stress disorder, was prosecuted for having attempted suicide. After ceasing to take his antidepressants, believing that they were causing seizures, he slashed his wrists. The Army prosecuted him for his 'self-injury', contending that his suicide attempt was 'prejudicial to good order and discipline' according to Article 134 of Army regulations. He was convicted, and sentenced to 180 days in jail, and given a dishonourable discharge. An appeals court eventually overturned the conviction, but the law may continue to be used as a disciplinary strategy for suicide attempts, which are deemed unacceptable in the military.

7.4 Why Punish Suicide Attempters?

Punishment may be perceived as having a utilitarian value in reducing crime or the repetition of an act that is not socially sanctioned. In the case of punishing suicide attempters, there are no empirical data supporting the belief that the threat of incarceration has a preventive effect. Overall, suicide rates are not lower in countries that have laws punishing attempters, despite the fact that reported suicides should be lower where suicide attempts are illegal, because of tendencies to underreport suicide mortality in places where suicide is viewed as unacceptable.

Punishments express the sentiments of the culture. As James Fitzjames Stephen stated (1883, cited in Kahan, 1996, p. 594): 'Laws give definite expression and solemn ratification ... to the hatred which is excited by the commission of an offence.' Expressive theories of punishment, which emphasise the value of punishment as venting or expressing moral condemnation, have been harshly criticised as being primitive in not considering the usefulness of such practices. However, others such as Kahan (1996) find value in expressive punishment, particularly because of the potential benefits of shaming the perpetrator.

Punishment of suicide attempters can also express the desire for retribution in order to do justice and punish a person who engages in a reprehensible or immoral act. If one believes that to take one's own life is tantamount to murdering another person and that it is not consequential that the life taken is that of the person engaging in the act, retribution may be seen as required. However, in order to justify retribution, it is assumed that the person engaged in a conscious act of will. This assumption, that suicide attempts are intentional acts, is complicated by the presumption, supported by scientific data (Mishara and Tousignant, 2004; World Health Organization, 2014), that people who attempt suicide generally suffer from a mental illness that compromises their ability to make rational or 'correct' choices. Liberal reactions in the main regard punishment of suicide attempters as a misplaced projection of societal anger towards people who engage in behaviours forbidden by widely accepted mores and/or religion.

Another aspect of punishment is its use to publicly shame a person who committed an offence, to express societal condemnation. A telling instance was the eighteenth-century practice in which the body of a person who died by suicide in Quebec, Canada, was dragged through the streets and displayed in a public place. Today, in many societies, the bodies of suicide victims are beaten or otherwise 'humiliated' and buried outside of cemetery grounds. Imprisonment for attempting suicide often reflects the desire to humiliate and shame by public affirmation both the person who engaged in the act and their family.

Kahan (1996, 2002) describes four contemporary shaming punishments: stigmatising publicity, literal stigmatisation (stamping the offender with a mark or symbol), self-abasement penalties, and condemnation. Punishment of suicide attempters can be considered stigmatising, as the attempter's status is publicised. Their punishment may also involve self-abasement as they are made to participate in a trial where their offence is described through a ritual of disgrace.

Public acts of contrition are not an essential part of the prosecution of offenders, although some may apologise during their trial for having attempted suicide. Kahan (2002) argues that the expression of condemnation is at least as important to shaming penalties as the infliction of the shame itself. Kahan argues that although there is little empirical evidence of the efficacy of shaming to deter repeated offences, shaming penalties express appropriate condemnation and may be effective and just deterrents. He contends that shaming sends a clear signal about what 'well-formed persons should and shouldn't [do]' and reinforces belief-dependent propensities to obey the law. He states that shaming penalties promote confidence in the law.

One may question the extent to which these justifications for shaming punishments apply to suicide attempters, who are likely to have a mental disorder; often attempt suicide while under the influence of alcohol or drugs, which compromise their ability to think about the consequences of their attempt; and whose risk of repeated attempts is more likely to be reduced by mental health treatment and psychosocial care than by fear of being shamed again after a repeat attempt.

Braithwaite (1989) believed that public shaming in general is useful since it helps create a shared moral conception of order. Massaro (1991) criticised this view, contending that law enforcement and judges are not family members ready to shun offenders, and thus are ineffective in inculcating cultural shame values. Massaro notes that anthropological studies suggest that the effectiveness of shaming as a method of norm enforcement depends upon whether the community also has rituals to redeem and reclaim the chastened offender afterwards.

For Massaro (1991), shaming requires witnesses who are considered to be important to the offender, and who, on learning of the shameful act, will condemn it. This results in fear of abandonment and rejection, which can have a dissuasive effect on potential perpetrators. Fear of shaming 'operates as a powerful sanction in most Mediterranean cultures, given the important role of honour and family' (Massaro, 1991, p. 1911). Until recently, the Mediterranean region has had suicide rates that were consistently lower than the world average. However, suicide rates have been increasing significantly in Italy and Greece following the recent economic crises, which indicates that the explanation of the effectiveness of shaming as a deterrent may be an ecological fallacy, where macro-level differences are fallaciously used to explain the behaviours of individuals.

According to Massaro (1991), shaming practices are most effective and meaningful when people fear that such practices will actually compromise the social standing of a member of a close-knit community. Massaro argues that 'if shaming ... [is] premised in inflated, ethnocentric, or otherwise inaccurate estimations of likely community responsiveness to public punishments, then they cannot produce the favourable outcomes that these reformers claim will occur' (Massaro 1991, p. 1928). Massaro concludes that shaming is ineffective in cultures such as the USA, where there is a lack of strong social norm cohesiveness and an absence of witnesses. Contemporary societies in the industrialised world also do not meet these criteria, particularly in urban cultures, where close-knit social integration is lacking. Braithwaite (1993) counters with the contention that although people living in a village are more vulnerable to shame by their neighbours than those in a city, twentieth-century city dwellers have a set of colleagues at work, in clubs, on parents' and citizen's committees, and in schools who can mobilise disapproval.

Social isolation is one of the prime vulnerability factors for a suicide attempt (Mishara and Tousignant, 2004; World Health Organization, 2014).

People at greatest risk have serious mental health problems that marginalise them from the potential sources of social shunning that Braithwaite enumerates. Furthermore, shunning is, in and of itself, a potent risk factor in already vulnerable populations.

The marginal status of suicide attempters in general, and the lack of indications of any preventive effects of punishment on the attempters, indicate that the shaming impact of laws that criminalise suicide attempts does not have favourable outcomes and may, by branding attempters further, inhibit help-seeking, the use of suicide prevention services, and mental health services.

7.5   Recommendations for Decriminalisation of Attempted Suicide

There is a need to promote the decriminalisation of suicide in the countries that have laws that treat suicide attempters as criminals rather than as people needing help for their mental health and related problems. Moreover, it would be useful to promote the adoption of a standardised definition of aiding, abetting, and assisting in suicide to develop more consistent laws and practices internationally. In some countries, the illegality of these activities is limited to minors; in others, only suicide pacts are illegal; and in some, the nature of the illegal acts is so broadly defined that inadvertent slights to people who attempt suicide may be interpreted as inciting their death. Furthermore, as the Internet is increasingly used to encourage people to attempt suicide and to provide information on suicide methods, laws and international jurisprudence need to address aiding and abetting suicide in cyberspace.

In those countries where decriminalisation has not and will not occur, it is still useful to develop strategies for giving mental health assistance to suicide attempters. Although religious and cultural values are important to respect, many countries have already successfully decriminalised suicide by promoting the belief that suicide attempters have not intentionally gone against dominant religious precepts and cultural values. This is buttressed by empirical evidence that recognises an attempter's pervasive inability to make an informed and competent decision (see the discussion of competency in Chapter 6). It is a reasonable assumption that the vast majority of suicide attempters need help and mental health services for their problems (World Health Organization, 2014). We conclude that in an overwhelming majority of cases it is most efficacious to treat suicidal behaviour as a psychosocial and mental health problem.

7.6   Moral Justifications of Criminal Penalties for Assisting, Inciting, and Encouraging Suicide

From moral and legal points of view, we continue to distinguish between the individual act of attempting suicide and the behaviour of assisting, inciting, or encouraging another person's suicidal behaviours. Even in jurisdictions where euthanasia or assisted suicide has been legalised for people who are terminally ill or who have interminable suffering, assisting in a suicide remains controversial. In responding to this reality, it is critical to differentiate instances when a person has a deteriorating or chronic physical illness from circumstances of psychological/emotional suffering.

Regardless of commitments to a specific set of values – religious beliefs, utilitarian-oriented social environmental perspectives, or Western liberal ones – there is a broad consensus that aiding and abetting suicide is morally unacceptable and should bring legal sanctions. In addressing the categories of perceived perpetrators who aid and abet a suicide, we should take care not to conflate a complicated set of actors who are variously motivated and reveal distinctive psychological profiles. In the case of assisted suicide of a terminally ill person who is experiencing interminable and insufferable pain, altruistic and compassionate reasons are likely present. However, others may have a personal gain from the suicide outcome, e.g., relatives who inherit or overburdened caregivers. In some situations, sadists may encourage suicide. It must be admitted that there are individuals who get pleasure in frequenting online forums to achieve their malevolent plans (see Chapter 4).

7.7   Conclusions

Despite the continuing trends towards repealing laws that make suicide a criminal offence, in 39 of the 193 countries of the world, laws or religious practices that have the force of law mandate punishment for suicidal behaviour. In many instances, the laws are rarely enforced, but each year people who have attempted suicide are jailed, rather than being provided with help for the mental health and psychosocial problems that led to their suicidal behaviour. Sometimes the laws are not enforced, but 'kept on the books', since politicians fear that repealing those laws would be interpreted as supporting behaviours that are condemned by the prevailing religion. In other countries, the enforcement of the laws is said to be justified by the belief, unsupported by research, that punishing suicide attempters will help prevent suicides. Countries that have repealed laws criminalising suicide have invariably had positive outcomes with increased access to mental health services for people with mental illness, increased public awareness of suicide prevention, and increased access to suicide prevention services.

8

· · · · · · ·

The Rhetoric of Assisted Suicide and Euthanasia ('Medical Assistance in Dying')

8.1   Introduction

In debates about euthanasia and assisted suicide, which are referred to as Medical Assistance in Dying (MAiD) in Canada, it is rare to find an article that begins with an expression of neutral interest and then proceeds to examine the various arguments and data before drawing conclusions based upon the results of a scholarly investigation. Although authors frequently give the impression of being impartial in their introduction, they invariably reach conclusions that matched their prior opinions. Positions tend to be clearly dichotomised: either one believes that the practice of euthanasia and assisted suicide is acceptable, or one believes that it is completely unacceptable in a just and moral society. Where there is some admission of a grey zone of uncertainty, authors attempt to persuade us that their beliefs are the only sensible way to resolve outstanding dilemmas.

Vehemently promoting a pro or con position may be useful when societies must decide to either legalise certain practices or not. Only a minority of countries or parts of countries have thus far accepted the legal practice of MAiD: Australia, Austria, Belgium, Canada, Colombia, Germany, Luxembourg, the Netherlands, New Zealand, Spain, Switzerland, and parts of the United States (USA: California, Colorado, Hawaii, Maine, Montana, New Jersey, New Mexico, Oregon, Vermont, Washington, and Washington, DC). However, in recent trends, scholarly articles mainly promote legalisation, to the point of recommending expansion of current practices. Is this a case of the philosophers and legislators being ahead of their time in promoting and rationalising the wave of the future? Alternatively, does the fact that only a small number of countries have legalised these practices indicate a substantial gap between the beliefs and desires of common citizens and the universe of those thinking in the abstracted realm? For the time being, what we do know is that each year more countries and states are debating MAiD, the legalisation of euthanasia, assisted suicide or both practices. Laws and legal practices vary greatly, and both ethical and empirical assessments of current practices are the subject of much controversy.

This chapter, which expands upon some of our earlier writings on this topic (Mishara and Weisstub, 2013), presents an examination of the premises and evidence in the rhetoric of MAiD. Inasmuch as any analysis cannot be totally impartial, we do not contend that our analysis is without influence from our experiences and philosophical affinities. Nonetheless, we summarise ethical arguments and available empirical data to offer some guidance to individuals who are involved in the development of policies and practices.

8.2 Threshold Vocabularies in Debates About Ending Life

The practices of MAiD are frequently confused with refusing treatment, withdrawing treatment, and the 'double effect'. The confusion has been exacerbated by the replacement of the terms 'euthanasia' and 'assisted suicide' by less-specific wording, such as MAiD. In Canada, euthanasia and assisted suicide has been legalised under the term MAiD ('Medical Assistance in Dying'). The image those words evoke, of a physician helping a person who is terminally ill, makes it easy to confound MAiD with providing palliative care to ease suffering, rather than clarifying that MAiD refers to intentionally ending a person's life.

Euthanasia involves an intentional act by a person (usually a physician) to end another person's life for compassionate reasons. The Canadian Senate's Special Committee on Euthanasia and Assisted Suicide defined euthanasia as 'the deliberate act undertaken by one person with the intention of ending the life of another person in order to relieve the person's suffering where the act is the cause of death' (Senate of Canada, 1995, p. 8). In countries where euthanasia is not legal, ending a person's life for whatever reason is considered homicide, although punishments depend on the circumstances, such as whether or not the intent was to harm or to kill. Assisted suicide is a specific type of suicide: killing oneself intentionally. Adding the word *assisted* to describe the suicide implies that another person assisted by providing the means, information about how to attempt suicide, or both (Mishara, 2002). In practice, assisted suicide generally involves providing lethal substances that one ingests to die. These practices differ from refusing treatment and withdrawing life-sustaining treatment, where a 'natural' death occurs without life being maintained by 'artificial' means.

The double-effect situation in regard to end-of-life practises occurs when a physician provides only sufficient medication to completely arrest the pain and suffering, but the effect of taking medication in sufficient quantities to stop suffering has the side effect of accelerating death. Double-effect reasoning follows from a long tradition that originated in the work of St Thomas Aquinas in the thirteenth century (Cavanaugh, 2006). Double-effect reasoning is used when the intended outcome is good (and thus morally justifiable), but one cannot realise the good outcome without also causing a foreseen but not intended bad effect. In double-effect reasoning, it is the morally justifiable intent and the accomplishment of the good outcome that counts. The secondary unintended harmful outcome is considered acceptable to attain the morally justified good result. In the case of a terminally ill person experiencing pain, control of pain and suffering is considered paramount, and controlling pain is justifiable even if life expectancy is compromised by the treatment, as long as the main intention of controlling pain is respected and no more medication is used than is required to attain an acceptable reduction in suffering. This practice requires that only enough medication to sufficiently control the pain and suffering is provided, so that life may be maintained as long as possible.

8.3 Legalisation of Euthanasia in Quebec as 'Medical Aid in Dying' (MAiD): Social Marketing and Legal Manoeuvring

On 10 June 2014, the province of Quebec in Canada adopted Bill 52 legalising euthanasia. The practice was called 'Medical Aid in Dying' (MAiD), which was defined as what is generally considered to be euthanasia: 'Care consisting of the administration of drugs or substances by a physician to a person at the end of life, at the person's request, with the goal of relieving his or her suffering by causing his or her death' (Assemblée nationale, 2014).

Legalising the practice of terminating a patient's life by a physician, even at that person's request, had appeared to be impossible within the Canadian legal context, at least at the time that Bill 52 was passed in Quebec in 2014 (Mishara and Weisstub, 2015). At that time there was a Conservative federal prime minister, who was against legalising euthanasia, and prior court cases had failed to determine that there was a 'right' to MAiD. After passage of Bill 52 in Quebec, the legal situation changed radically when the Supreme Court of Canada, on 6 February 2015, rendered a judgement in the case of *Carter v. Canada* (Attorney General), which legalised the practice of assisted suicide and/or euthanasia throughout Canada (Supreme Court Judgements, 2015-02-06).

At the time Bill 52 was passed, it seemed clear that federal laws prohibiting taking another person's life under any circumstances would render it impossible to legalise the taking of a life by a physician for compassionate reasons anywhere in Canada. Federal law (Criminal Code of Canada, sections 14 and 241 (b)) specifically stated: 'It is unlawful to take another person's life and one cannot use as a justification for taking a life the fact that the person wanted to be killed.' Similarly, federal criminal Law 241(b) made it a criminal act to aid and abet in a suicide, which would seem to render it illegal to engage in assisted suicide regardless of the context. The Quebec Law legalised euthanasia but did not allow assisted suicide. One may wonder how this provincial law could be justified, given the explicit prohibitions in the Federal Criminal Code.

Although criminal adjudication of killing is governed by federal law, the provinces in Canada have relative autonomy in regulating medical care provided to residents of their province. By characterising killing a person as being part of a range of medical interventions to 'help' patients who are suffering, Bill 52 asserted the province's role in health care and its assumed 'right' to legalise ending the life of a patient as being a health-care activity, which is under its provincial jurisdiction. However, the use of the terminology 'Medical Assistance in Dying' to describe the practice of euthanasia also served a second political purpose: It helped foster support for the bill by not explicitly informing the general public about the exact nature of what was being legalised.

Marcoux *et al.* (2007) found that in Quebec, Canada, before the practice was legalised under the rubric of MAiD, 70% of the population favoured legalisation of MAiD. However, in delving into the matter further, Marcoux *et al.* (2007) found that over two thirds of the population was unable to identify whether vignettes depicted end-of-life practises correctly, and they often thought that legalising MAiD meant legalising other practices, such as refusing or stopping treatment, that were already legal in Quebec. The more people were confused about the nature of euthanasia and other end-of-life practises, the greater the likelihood they would be in favour of legalisation of MAiD. After passage of Bill 52, Marcoux *et al.* (2015) conducted another survey, this time of Quebec's physicians and nurses, asking them about what was currently legal and illegal, as well as what practices were legalised by Bill 52. They found that 46% wrongly thought that it was not permitted to withdraw a potentially life-prolonging treatment at the patient's request and that only 40% believed that the practice of MAiD, as legalised by Bill 52, permitted the use of lethal medication to end a patient's life.

More recently, six years after legalisation of the practice of providing medical assistance in dying in Quebec, an interview study in Quebec found that 65% of respondents confused MAiD with other legal forms of end-of-life practises, such as palliative care, withdrawing and withholding life-sustaining treatments, and advance directives for treatment (Plaisance *et al.*, 2022). Although there were generally quite favourable attitudes towards MAiD, there was so much confusion in what constitutes MAiD that the authors concluded that it was not the legalised 'MAiD' practises of euthanasia and assisted suicide that people supported.

There is a long history of using euphemisms to describe the practice of killing in order to render practices palatable that otherwise might be viewed with disfavour if they had been precisely defined. When a bomb targeting an enemy combatant also kills innocent men, women, and children, this is often described as 'collateral damage'. The eugenics movement in the early part of the twentieth century used scientific terminology and positive slogans to describe as 'beneficial' what eventually developed into the mass extermination of millions of people.

Bill 52, rather than explicitly stating that euthanasia was to be rendered legal, indicated that what was legalised was 'medical aid in dying'. The use of this terminology resulted in mass public support. Who can be against getting help from a physician when dying? Few people actually read the legislation, and it is likely that many people failed to understand, as was the case for 58% of physicians in the province after passage of the law, that 'medical aid in dying' is defined in Quebec as ending a person's life at their request, which is the standard definition of euthanasia (Marcoux *et al.*, 2015).

Is there an ethical imperative for lawmakers to clearly inform the public about the explicit nature of what is being legalised, particularly when the law in question concerns permitting physicians to end people's lives? In

Quebec, the legalisation of the practice of euthanasia was supported by a majority of the population, at least to the extent that Quebecers said they were in favour of 'medical aid in dying'. Calling euthanasia 'MAiD' effectively served to sanitise the practice morally. In essence, this is effective social marketing. Selling ideas, as with selling products, consists of giving the impression that the product is highly desirable. Is using political persuasion and rhetoric justified in convincing or placating the general population for a just cause? What are the ethical responsibilities of legislators in this regard?

When there is real consensus that to preserve a social priority, such as democracy, the risk of loss of life is considered appropriate or ethical; there can be a 'just' or justifiable war. In this way, sacrifices are justified, and violence is legitimised. But where an individual life is at issue, and its preservation is clouded by economic exigencies and limited access to alternatives such as palliative or hospice care, what are the legitimate burdens to be placed on legislators to ensure that the public is fully informed about the procedures and values at stake? We submit that the provision of alternative means of alleviating the suffering that may lead to a request for MAiD should be required before we grant such requests.

8.4   The Constitutional Sword: A Double-Edged Conundrum

It is notable that theological arguments have rarely been in the forefront of recent debates on euthanasia and assisted suicide. Constitutional guarantees are generally invoked as both the justification for legalising MAiD and as the justification for forbidding these practices. Constitutional guarantees of freedom and non-discrimination are often cited as reasons for legalisation. Choosing the manner, time, and place of one's death has been described as a simple exercise of individual freedom of choice. However, legalisation goes beyond simply allowing people to choose. Over and above accepting that people may choose to die, legalisation involves either providing the means to kill oneself, as is the case in assisted suicide, or actually having a third party intervene to end a person's life, as with euthanasia.

There are multiple motivations for providing MAiD. To begin with, one can contend that without proper medical help, people may botch their suicide attempt, potentially leading to either suffering a horrific death or not dying, with the accompanying risk of becoming permanently handicapped.

In Canada, constitutional arguments have been made that there is an inherent inequity in the case of the severely handicapped – for example, in reference to the paralysis that occurs in the advanced stages of certain degenerative diseases. People with severe handicaps may be viewed as being unable to exercise the 'right' to suicide because of their illness. Providing euthanasia could be seen as the state fulfilling an obligation to make access to medical treatment as equal as possible for all citizens, providing everyone with an effective 'choice to die'. The obvious counterargument is that the state does not have a responsibility to provide citizens the means to realise all of their desires, particularly for the act of ending one's life.

In countries where euthanasia has been legalised, almost all those who die in this manner are fully capable of suicide. It is a rare exception that people requesting MAiD are truly incapable of executing the act. Cases of advanced paralysis are in fact rare. In the Netherlands, the majority of euthanasia cases involve people suffering from cancer (91.1%), and fewer than 6.4% have a neurological disorder that may result in loss of motor control, with euthanasia administered while the patient is still capable of assisted suicide (Regional Euthanasia Review Committees, 2020). In Belgium, 65.5% of people who died by euthanasia suffered from cancer and 8.7% had degenerative neurological disorders (Commission fédérale de Contrôle et d'Évaluation de l'Euthanasie, 2020). In addition, there is only a moderate relationship between the desire to die and the presence of physical handicaps. The desire to die is mediated by other factors, such as perceived burdensomeness, depressive symptoms, having a physical disability, and pain (Khazem, 2018; Mishara, 1999b).

Constitutional guarantees of freedom are also used as an argument against legalising euthanasia and assisted suicide. It can be argued that the state has an obligation to protect its citizens, particularly the most vulnerable, to enable life (Finlay and George, 2011; Hawryluck, 2017; Herring, 2022). Governments often intervene to protect citizens from self-harm, requiring them to wear seatbelts and motorcycle helmets and disallowing the purchase of harmful drugs. In both euthanasia and assisted suicide, this protection can be fulfilled through prioritising palliative care and psychosocial interventions before MAiD is deemed an option. MAiD advocates contend that the fundamental societal obligation to enhance and preserve life is superseded by unbearable, unavoidable physical or psychological suffering. Some secular constitutionalists contend that society must make a valiant effort to provide palliative care in all circumstances and that this is generally sufficient to significantly reduce pain and suffering.

Finally, we must ask ourselves whether we should show our support for the right to life in the face of possible transgressions by maintaining legal sanctions against all acts of MAiD. A middle-ground position is that there should be carefully construed permissions when people in extreme suffering have evidenced independence and voluntariness.

In contemporary Western countries, judges, as responsible decision-makers, are often fearful to let go of their guardianship role as the paramount protectors of the right to life (Starck, 2002). However, in the face of instances of overwhelming human suffering, and imbued with contemporary values of 'autonomy' and 'self-determination', judges and legislative authorities seek avenues to express humane compassion towards competent citizens whose suffering has become unbearable. Once we have made any exception to the primacy of protecting life for such cases, surveillance becomes necessary to protect against inappropriate and expanding exceptions and the misuse of professional discretion.

In judicial opinions, Western civil and common-law systems reiterate the commitment to the right to life. Clearly defined exceptions have been based on defences of bodily integrity, war conditions, or punishments for heinous crimes against humanity. Judges have had to deal with requests from individuals and intensive lobbying, and they have attempted to balance the weight of historical commitments with constitutional principles.

Overall, the preponderance of judicial opinions indicates that judges in common-law jurisdictions who had been defensive in accommodating requests for euthanasia and assisted suicide based on personal autonomy, are increasingly being called upon to consider a 'right' to MAiD.

The situation in Canada is a case in point. In *Rodriguez v. British Columbia* (Judgements of the Supreme Court of Canada, 1993), the Supreme Court of Canada emphasised that although Sue Rodriguez, who was suffering from amyotrophic lateral sclerosis (ALS), also known as Lou Gehrig's disease, made a compelling request, the Canadian Charter of Rights and Freedoms superseded any right to assisted suicide. The court's decision prohibited assisted suicide entirely, in order to defend the rights of vulnerable populations.

British and American higher court decisions had essentially followed the spirit of the *Rodriguez* ruling. The British House of Lords pronounced that not only was there an absence of a right to assisted suicide in the tradition of common law, but, like the Canadian Charter, the European Convention on Human Rights provides no guaranteed right to assisted suicide. In addressing Article 2 of the European Convention, dealing with the right to life, the European Court of Human Rights followed *Rodriguez* (1993) and *Pretty v. United Kingdom* (2002). There have been some exceptions to this in subsequent decisions in the United Kingdom (On the application of *Purdy v. Director of Public Prosecutions*, 2009), articulating that where a set of conditions has been met that documents the goodwill of the alleged perpetrator, discretion is permitted concerning whether or not to proceed with prosecution.

In Canada, the Supreme Court decided in 2015 that sections of the Criminal Code (sections 241(b) and 14) that prohibited assisted death infringed upon Section 7 of the Canadian Charter, which guarantees the right to life, liberty, and security of the person, and that those sections are not in accordance with principles of fundamental justice:

> An individual's response to a grievous and irremediable medical condition is a matter critical to their dignity and autonomy. The prohibition denies people in this situation the right to make decisions

concerning their bodily integrity and medical care and thus impinges upon their liberty. And by leaving them to endure intolerable suffering, it impinges on their security of the person (*Carter v. Canada* (Attorney General)).

In response to that decision, the Canadian Parliament passed Bill C-14 in 2016 to allow euthanasia and assisted suicide, together called Medical Assistance in Dying (MAiD), for people whose natural death is 'reasonably foreseeable'.

In 2019, the Superior Court of Quebec, in *Truchon c. Procureur general du Canada* (QCCS 3792) determined that the requirement that death be 'reasonably foreseeable' in order to access MAiD was contrary to the right of equality. Neither the government of Quebec nor the government of Canada appealed that decision. In response to that decision, in 2021 the Criminal Code was amended again by Bill C-7 to allow individuals with a 'grievous and irremediable medical condition', but whose natural death is not reasonably foreseeable, to access MAiD, with the stipulation that people whose sole medical condition that is grievous and irremediable is a mental disorder would not have access to MAiD until March 2023.

After controversies developed concerning proceeding with expanding MAiD to people with a mental disorder as the sole illness associated with the request, in March 2023 Bill C-39 was adopted to grant a one-year delay in the access to MAiD for people with a mental disorder, until 17 March 2024.

At the time this book went to press, there was heated debate in Canada over the adequacy of safeguards in the current MAiD laws to protect vulnerable people from dying prematurely, rather than receiving treatment for their suffering. Furthermore, proposals for further expansion of access to MAiD were recommended. In February 2023, the Special Joint Committee on Medical Assistance in Dying (2023), whose members had a majority appointed by the ruling liberal government that explicitly promoted expansion of MAiD, completed its statutory review of the MAiD laws. The Canadian Parliamentary Committee held public hearings in which there was testimony from vehement proponents for an expansion of access to MAiD to respect the autonomy of anyone suffering intolerably from a chronic illness, and equally vehement pleas for protecting vulnerable populations of people with disabilities and mental disorders, demanding improved access to treatment, rather than easier access to MAiD.

The committee report made 23 recommendations to parliament on five topics: the state of palliative care in Canada, protections for Canadians with disabilities, MAiD for mental disorders as a sole underlying medical condition, MAiD for mature minors, and advance requests for MAiD.

Forty-six people, expert on the five topics, who had testified before the committee as expert witnesses, including researchers and representatives of major organisations that defend the rights of people with disabilities and people with mental illness, submitted a brief to the members of parliament (Chochinov *et al.*, 2023). They contended in the brief that the committee report ignored much of the input by the recognised experts who expressed concern and caution.

The 46 experts wrote that the report misconstrued, minimised, and completely ignored key evidence to protect Canadians. They concluded that the recommendations failed to provide Canadians with the safeguards necessary to prevent wrongful death, subjecting large segments of the Canadian population to potential harms.

The critics expressed concerns about all 23 recommendations. Key examples of disagreements included whether palliative care should be a prerequisite to access MAiD. This counter-position noted that palliative care is not available for the majority of Canadians. Only 21% have contact with palliative care services, usually in the two weeks before receiving MAiD. Polls show that most Canadians prioritise expanding palliative care over expanding access to MAiD (Angus Reid Institute, 2023).

The critics thought the recommendation to allow prisoners who request to die by MAiD be allowed to leave prison for palliative care in preparation for MAiD could incite prisoners to opt for MAiD as a way of being able spend time outside prison before dying. The opponents insisted for a right to palliative care while in prison without having to first request MAiD.

When the requirement that death be 'foreseeable' was eliminated from the MAiD requirements, all persons with a disability became eligible for MAiD; disability was thereby conflated with suffering. The critics insisted that it is more humanely responsible that people with disabilities have access to affordable housing and support to live in the community.

The parliamentary committee report stated that not allowing MAiD for persons with a mental disorder as the sole underlying medical condition (MD- SUMC) would be discriminatory. Opponents have claimed that providing MAiD to persons with MD-SUMC would be the ultimate form of discrimination by exposing marginalised individuals to avoidable deaths based on faulty assessments by evaluators, wrongly reporting that an individual's mental illness was 'irremediable'. We have already noted that research indicates that it is impossible to assess when the suffering from a mental disorder is irremediable, or indeed to distinguish between a request for MAiD and suicidality. Suicidal thoughts are often symptoms of inadequately treated mental disorders.

Furthermore, expanding access to MAiD for mature minors (without any minimum age) ignores scientific evidence that children and teenagers do not have fully developed abilities for risk assessment and mature decision-making. The parliamentary committee further recommended that when minors request MAiD, 'where appropriate, the parents or guardians of a mature minor be consulted in the course of the assessment process for MAiD, but that the will of a minor who is found to have requisite decision-making capacity ultimately takes priority' (Committee Recommendation 19). Others have viewed such a policy as undermining the ability of parents to protect children, going against existing provisions for parental consent to treatment.

The last section of the parliamentary committee report concerns recommendations to allow advance consent to MAiD, so that people may plan to have their lives ended by MAiD. Critics have cited evidence of the 'disability paradox', namely that people tend to have a much more negative perception of their quality of life prior to becoming disabled than afterwards. Furthermore, there are no data to confirm that written advance directives predict future wishes accurately. Advance consent is not fully informed in the way that contemporaneous consent is. It cannot be withdrawn once the person is incapable, thus violating the Convention on the Rights of Persons with Disabilities (United Nations, 2006).

In response to the controversies concerning proceeding with expanding MAiD to people with a mental disorder as the sole illness associated with the request, in March 2023 Bill C-39 was adopted in Canada to grant a one-year delay in the access to MAiD for people with a mental disorder, until 17 March 2024. However, the bill did not provide for any further review of the original decision to expand access to people with a mental disorder or any modifications to the criteria for access to MAiD, such as a requirement for a psychiatric evaluation, for persons requesting MAiD for their suffering from a mental disorder. If no new legislation is passed, in 2024 people whose suffering is only from a mental disorder will have access to MAiD.

A fundamental issue in the ongoing debate is the determination of what constitutes an ethical basis for determining access to MAiD. On the one hand, there are activists who believe that access to MAiD should be available with a minimum of constraints, allowing people to decide how and when they shall die. Proponents of allowing a maximum of autonomy in choosing MAiD believe that to limit MAiD risks discriminating against people with different forms of suffering and different causes of their desire to die. Critics are concerned that death as a treatment for suffering must only be a last resort, and the alleviation of suffering should be the priority in order to ensure that MAiD does not become a substitute for care and support.

8.5   Autonomy: An Intense and Elusive Value

Arguably, privacy was a key focus of bioethics in the 1970s and 1980s, concerning access to reproductive rights and a need for protection against the intrusion of governments into the 'bedrooms of the nation' (in the words of Pierre Elliot Trudeau, former Prime Minister of Canada). Autonomy appears to be a major bio-ethical focus of the early decades of the twenty-first century. This is not surprising. The political consciousness regarding the experiences of women and minorities have made exponential leaps in recent decades. This has resulted in the value of autonomy coming to be associated with the assertion of self in the public arena, and the promotion of autonomous decision-making has been a primary argument for the legalisation and expansion of MAiD.

Autonomy has been associated with our sense of identity. It can be viewed as a reaction against paternalism and the governance of our lives by elites, and a rejection of colonial or Victorian values. Autonomy has been personified as a basic value for all human beings, the value without which we cannot speak meaningfully about humans acting in a free world. It is on the tongue of liberation movements of all descriptions.

The hard questions concern how to clearly define autonomy and how it functions in the universe of practical ethics. Jonathan Herring (2022), who has written thoughtfully on the components of suicide and its relation to autonomy, has concluded:

> The extent to which a decision is autonomous is variable, [and] opens up a more flexible approach, allowing autonomy to be weighed against the degree of harm. It is where the harm is serious that we need to take considerable care in determining what precisely it is that the patient wants and only accede to their wishes where there is a strongly autonomous decision to die. (Herring, 2022, pp. 95–96)

Herring rates autonomy on a scale from high to low. When the issue at hand is serious, such as suicide or death by MAiD, he contends that it should be permitted only if the level of autonomy is high. Decisions of a trivial or less-important nature can be made less autonomously. In doing so, impulsive decisions are set aside. According to Professor Herring, weakly autonomous decisions invite interventions, whereas highly autonomous decisions do not.

For which people do we respect choices enough to not intervene in their suicide attempt? Would it be an existentialist and creative author such as Camus, a public intellectual and distinguished philosopher of US Constitutional values, a president of the Hemlock Society, or even a student who sets herself on fire to protest against global imperfections or cruelties such as climate change or instances of torture? Herring understands that most suicides are either done in haste or connected to feelings of low self-esteem, hopelessness, lack of belonging, etc.

How much significance can we give to the idea that autonomy is inherently connected to a set of values, an enriched view of looking at the world, which represents a mature self-image? Furthermore, much of modern society sets itself aside from communal thinking – that is, from responsibility to family or extended groups.

8.6   Legalism and Autonomy

The legalist approach, which emphasises adherence to laws, has been represented by many statutes specifically dealing with capacity, consent, and autonomy. Suicide is the most sensitive area for the application of the existing laws. Many cases are judged under the mental capacity legislation found in countries all over the world.

It is interesting to look at the legalistic capacity criteria, perhaps the most referred-to example being the MacArthur Competence Assessment Tool for Treatment (MacCAT-T), which is the most widely used instrument by mental health professionals in North America. However, when we look at the actual criteria (Grisso *et al.*, 1997), it is essentially a high bar asking if individuals can understand the information about their illness and the probable consequences of treatment; it evaluates their ability to reason.

If, on the other hand, we turn to more empathetic and compassionate criteria, a more 'humanistic approach', linking the person to a history of relations with family, friends, and a host of 'narratives' (Barrett *et al.*, 2022; Mackenzie and Stoljar, 2000), how realistically could that be implemented? With what group of experts and with what balance of risk, harm, and autonomy? There is already a financial challenge in the application of legalistic criteria linked to the costs of involving professionals, hospitals, clinics, and governments to fulfil the promise of explicitly ethically sensitive standards. It is unlikely that the techniques associated with Narrative Ethics will prove to be useful in suicide prevention. Life histories are generally considered to be an intrinsic component of clinical assessments of suicide risk. However, narrative ethics associated techniques may have relevance for MAiD, where the application of a small number of legal criteria for access may benefit from understanding the life history of the individual.

The legalists who are committed to a low bar will defend their position by insisting that documenting capacity is the best that can be done, apart from very special cases and conditions, which are highly exceptional. (See Section 8.4 of Chapter 8 for a more detailed discussion of capacity.)

In current discussions about medically assisted dying, how we see autonomy, how we relate it to capacity, and how we understand the infirmities of those who choose MAiD will determine the priority given to high or low autonomy in the world of bioethics. Finally, practical ethics must benefit from turning to credible human situations to see how legal criteria play out in real life.

8.7   Human Dignity

It is most probably a safe assumption that if we were to search for a consensus across cultures, we would find widespread fear about dying in a degraded or undignified manner (Etinson, 2020). Contemporary empirical research with respect to 'dignity in terminally ill patients' has attempted to quantify 'dignity' and develop dignity-assessment inventories, examining qualities such as symptom distress, existential distress, dependency, peace of mind, and social support (Bagnasco *et al.*, 2020; Chochinov *et al.*, 2008).

Dignity can be seen as the highest value in advanced constitutional cultures. Human dignity is at the forefront of declarations of human rights and constitutions. Groups that affirm self-assertiveness have found agreement on the matter of our responsibility as a society to strive for a dignified death. From a philosophical standpoint, since there are extreme divergences about what that should entail, there is a challenge to clarify human dignity as a concept (Choo *et al.*, 2020, Shultziner, 2007).

The social liberal ideal is that each individual is possessed of an inherent dignity: that human dignity at once represents the individualistic morality brought on by the Enlightenment, which defers to the notions of autonomy and respect for people, while attending to a social dimension of humanity where people are given a special status of protection that goes to the very core of what it means to be a person, with all that it implies (Thomasma and Weisstub, 2004).

In earlier historical periods, human dignity seemed to be an aristocratic attribute and was at odds with more modern – or indeed, liberal – expressions. Consequently, it may be that our understanding of dignity inevitably has a confusing component, as we have an unwitting tendency to relate dignity to the dignified behaviour or social style of those in high-ranking social positions.

Notwithstanding this complicated history, human dignity has become a truly central value within many Western cultures. Even though there has been considerable cynicism expressed by legal philosophers and social theorists about the meaning of dignity, liberal thinkers have tended to treat human dignity as an overarching protector value (Dupre, 2009). As an idealised primal right, human dignity may be the most suitable value on which to found a judicial system, a key reference point to defend respect for personhood.

The question remains whether human dignity, apart from an idealised statement about respect for humanity, carries with it an internal logic that allows us to clarify its relationship to other fundamental values. The bioethicist Ruth Macklin (1999, p. 1419) has stated, 'Is dignity a useful concept for an ethical analysis of medical activities? A close inspection of leading examples shows that appeals to dignity are either vague restatements of other, more precise notions, or mere slogans that add nothing to an understanding of the topic.' The issue remains: whether dignity can provide direction about how to deal with conflicting values when decisions have to be made to ensure that people in vulnerable states can make clear individual choices – for example, about the manner in which they wish to end their lives (Dupre, 2009; Foster, 2019).

At the outset, what we should admit is that human dignity colours differently depending both upon the social and individual needs in question (Choo *et al.*, 2020; Weisstub and Thomasma, 2001). Is it the case that its centrality and attractiveness for global ethics – and indeed, for medical ethics – may be its malleability rather than the tightness of its logic?

The human need for a dignified death is grounded in a psychological longing or drive to be treated as a human being and not as an expendable commodity. Another way of putting this is that a wish to be honoured by one's family, friendship circle, health professionals, and society itself is fundamental to the human species. If you look at dignity in this way, it may be that honour and dignity are interchangeable expressions of this primal need or drive.

We might even suggest that honour could replace dignity as an expression of this need. When dignity is taken away from a rights vocabulary and is turned into a language of universal human needs, perhaps it is better understood as approximating the concept of honour.

Both dignity and honour can be associated with a process of recognising the 'other'. This recognition brings us to a covenantal relation where differences of power are recognised, but obligations flow morally from the unique commitments that are part of the relationship, whether between God and people or between medical professionals and their patients (Nahme and Feller, 2024).

Honour in its pre-modern incarnation was undoubtedly shackled by pomp and status. However, if we look early in Western human history at '*kavod*', found in the biblical commandment to honour one's father and mother, we can locate honour as a sustaining force of mutuality (Weiner, 2022). Perhaps this is more compelling than 'dignitas', which in its historical Western evolution has been more linked to worthiness or attributes deserving of our social respect. In any event, whether honour sounds a deeper moral chord or at this point is interchangeable with dignity as a reference for respecting the vulnerable, they are jointly useful for facilitating untrammelled and free choices to make about one's life. They are viable tools for empowering individuals making profoundly personal decisions. We should agree that honour and dignity equally could connect to respect, concern, and even mutuality. Perhaps we could also conclude that concern about the choice of words should give way to the more pressing question of how to concretely protect people found in situations of vulnerability.

8.8   Shoring Up the Slippery Slope

It is clear that there has been an expansion of threshold eligibility for euthanasia and assisted suicide in the Netherlands, Canada, and Switzerland, and Belgium as well. Courts in the Netherlands have upheld the right of people who are mentally ill, but have no physical ailments, to have access to euthanasia or assisted suicide to alleviate intolerable suffering. Canada is set to do likewise in March 2024, unless new legislation is passed beforehand.

The systematic review by Calati *et al.* (2021) of assisted suicide and euthanasia in psychiatric patients was based upon research from the Netherlands, Belgium, and Switzerland. The review concluded that research indicates that people who die by assisted suicide or euthanasia in these countries have characteristics 'very similar to traditional suicides'. They felt that there is a need to revise the criteria for access to euthanasia and assisted suicide to focus on unbearable suffering, decision capacity, and possibilities for improvement of their mental well-being.

In the Netherlands, Belgium, and Canada, the criteria of unbearable and irremediable suffering can be used to access death by euthanasia or by assisted suicide, without the requirement that the person suffer from a terminal or degenerative illness, and without clearly distinguishing between physical and mental suffering (Dees *et al.*, 2010), although people with only a mental illness will not have access in Canada until 2024. Alacreu-Crespo *et al.* (2020) pointed out that unbearable psychological suffering in those countries was both a criterion allowing access to euthanasia or assisted suicide and an indication of the need for suicide prevention interventions in daily practice. They cite research findings that psychological pain and depression may compromise decision-making abilities. Furthermore, as Verhofstadt *et al.* (2017) indicated, although patients may experience their suffering as irremediable, often the major factors associated with their suffering are economic or resource-access issues, which could change their situation and wishes.

In Switzerland, there have been cases of assisted suicide justified on the basis that the person suffered from an intolerable mental disorder (Calati *et al.*, 2021, Levene and Parker, 2011). In that country, assisted suicide can be practised by laypeople, in some instances on psychiatric patients, including inpatients while in psychiatric care (Frei *et al.*, 2001).

In the Netherlands, an earlier study found that each year approximately 400 people request euthanasia or physician-assisted suicide in the absence of a severe physical or mental disease. These patients are primarily elderly and, according to a survey of 408 Dutch health-care professionals (Rurup *et al.*, 2005), the main reasons for the requests (not mutually exclusive) were 'being through with life' (55%), physical decline associated with ageing (55%), and 'being tired of life' (48%). Although most of those requests were denied on the basis of the patient not suffering 'unbearably' and 'hopelessly' or the patient not suffering from a severe disease, 3% of all general practitioners surveyed said that they had granted a request for euthanasia or assisted suicide to a patient who did not suffer from a severe physical or psychiatric disease.

Since unbearable and hopeless suffering is a criterion for access to physician-assisted death according to the Dutch Euthanasia Act, it is concerning to recognise the extent to which subjective interpretations of what constitutes 'unbearable and hopeless suffering' can play a role in evaluations by physicians for access to premature death. In the aforementioned study (Rurup *et al.*, 2005), although 38% of patients who requested euthanasia were characterised by the physician who received the request as having symptoms of melancholia or depression, most were not provided with treatment. Of those who received treatment, half later withdrew or modified their request for MAiD.

There are data from the Netherlands indicating that euthanasia is sometimes practised in the absence of a request from the patient, generally in the last days of life when the person is unconscious and unable to participate in the decision that life be terminated. For example, Onwuteaka-Philipsen *et al.* (2012), found 13 cases of ending life in 2010 without an explicit request by a patient, 24 cases in 2005, and 42 cases in 2001. A study by Smets *et al.* (2012) in Belgium asked physicians to identify whether different end-of-life practises should be classified as euthanasia and reported, in accordance with the 2002 law legalising euthanasia. They found that 19% of the physicians did not identify terminating a patient's life by injecting a neuromuscular relaxant as a case of euthanasia, and 27% did not know that it should be reported. Only 21% of the physicians correctly identified a case of euthanasia with morphine as being euthanasia. This evidence indicates that legalisation of euthanasia and the development of standards for its use does not eliminate such illegitimate practices. Research shows that there are transgressions in countries that have legalised euthanasia or assisted suicide. The response by supporters is invariably the same: there are probably more 'questionable' practices in countries where all foreshortening of life is illegal. However, there are no empirical data to back up this contention.

8.9   Towards a Best-Policy Model

'*On ne peut pas être contre la vertu*': 'One cannot be against virtue.' This applies to views of hospice and palliative care to treat pain and suffering that meet the psychological needs of people suffering from a grave or terminal illness. Everyone is in favour of providing access to good palliative care. However, in most countries palliative care is available only for a minority of citizens, and usually only near the end of life, when all interventions to prolong life have failed. There are a number of reasons that patients do not receive palliative care even when it is available. Many simply do not know enough to ask, sometimes assuming that their suffering or feeling depressed is 'normal' under the circumstances and there is not much that can be done about it. Without a specially trained palliative care team, patients may not be receiving good-quality care because their physician was not well trained in pain management and in meeting the psychological needs of patients. Patients sometimes refuse palliative care and ask for MAiD instead because of a lack of clear understanding of what palliative care involves. The patient may simply prefer to die rather than continue living with this form of help. There are also financial considerations: some patients prefer to die sooner so that their assets will not be taken to cover the expensive costs of prolonged care and be preserved for their heirs. Also, in many jurisdictions, palliative care is not available to a substantial proportion of the population.

It is important to note that palliative care is generally cheaper than 'care as usual'. People now often spend the last days of their life in hospitals. In Canada 45% of individuals die in hospitals, and treatment as a hospital patient is costly (Bekelman *et al.*, 2016; Tung *et al.*, 2018). A US study found that hospice use reduced medical expenditures by 25% during the last year of life, an average saving of $2,309 per hospice user (Taylor *et al.*, 2007).

The Office of the Parliamentary Budget Officer (2020) in Canada assessed the financial impact of MAiD in 2021, before MAiD was expanded to include people for whom death is not 'reasonably foreseeable' (Bernier *et al.*, 2020). They reported that after deducting the costs of administering MAiD, the provincial governments saved $86.9 million because of savings associated with the reduction in the period of time people lived due to the availability of MAiD. The report was requested by a senator preceding the adoption of Bill C-7, which expanded MAiD to people for whom death was not reasonably foreseeable. As requested by the senator, they estimated the additional savings in health costs from expanding access to MAiD to be $62 million, with a total reduction in costs of $149 million per year. The report estimated that the total number of people dying by MAiD would be 7,629 in 2021. However, the actual number in Canada for 2021 was 10,064,

32% greater than estimated, resulting in an estimated saving of $196.68 million, with increasing savings annually as the proportion of Canadians dying by MAiD continues to increase.

It is impossible to determine the extent to which savings in end-of-life health costs may play a role in legalisation and expansion of access to MAiD in different countries. In Canada, universal access to government-sponsored health care is provided to all residents. In countries where patients and their families must pay for health care, and where sufficient funding for universal health care is not available, the cost savings from MAiD could be a consideration, and the financial burden upon families to remain alive may be an important motivation for seeking MAiD.

8.10 Euthanasia and Assisted Suicide: Ethical and Practical Distinctions

Are there ethical or important practical distinctions between the practice of euthanasia and assisted suicide? In the USA, assisted suicide has been legalised in several states, but there has been little discussion of also legalising euthanasia. In Belgium and Luxembourg, euthanasia is the practice and, in Canada and the Netherlands, although both assisted suicide and euthanasia are legally available, euthanasia performed by physicians is the predominant practice. In Switzerland, assisted suicide was never formally legalised; however, it can be practised because there never were any laws rendering the practice illegal.

As presented in Chapter 1, one of the most common characteristics of suicide is ambivalence on the part of suicidal individuals. Only a tiny proportion of people who seriously consider suicide will attempt suicide (Evans *et al.*, 2017; Mishara and Tousignant, 2004). Even people who die by suicide have some level of ambivalent feelings, and a part of them would like to continue to live, despite their great suffering. It is reported by suicide prevention workers that most survivors are grateful to be alive (Cleary, 2019).

In Chapter 1, we emphasised that the majority of seriously suicidal individuals change their mind and find ways of solving or living with their problems. The small proportion of suicide attempters who die from their attempts (less than 1 in 50) is not due to an extreme inability of humans to end their lives. It can be explained by the fact that most people, after they have initiated a suicide attempt, change their minds and stop the attempt or try to get help if they are able.

Proponents of MAiD invariably ignore the issue of ambivalent feelings, usually explaining without evidence that the presence of an interminable degenerative illness and impending death results in more certainty in decisions to accelerate death. In the preceding Chapter we indicated that 34% of people in Oregon, USA, who obtained lethal medications for assisted suicide, changed their minds and never used the medication. Assisted suicide as practised in the USA allows for the exercise of the individual's right to change their mind.

When euthanasia is practised instead of assisted suicide, a doctor administers the lethal substance at an appointed time. In this somewhat depersonalised situation, where the busy doctor believes the person 'should die' and is ready to act right then and there, it is less easy for the patient to express ambivalence. Unlike the situation with assisted suicide in Oregon, patients who make an appointment for euthanasia rarely do not die on the appointed day. In Switzerland, where non-profit organisations provide the lethal medication that is administered by their employee, in their facility, and at a predetermined time, there have been few reports of people changing their mind (Calati *et al.*, 2021).

8.11   Rational Suicide: Between Logic and Reality

In Chapter 1, we contended that most important human decisions are not reasonable; important human decision-making has highly emotionally charged components that are influenced by social expectations and can easily cast reason aside. The requirements for access to euthanasia and assisted suicide do not account for the irrationality of human decision-making. The typical criteria for providing access to death to a patient is that the person has interminable and unsupportable suffering. Research on human decision-making suggests that when a person is experiencing pain, decision-making becomes less rational (Apkarian *et al.*, 2004; Higgins *et al.*, 2018).

This results in the paradoxical situation where proponents of legalising euthanasia and assisted suicide insist upon patients having the right to make a 'rational' choice under circumstances where rational decision-making is much less likely to occur. This is a serious challenge for physicians, who must determine whether to accept a request for euthanasia or assisted suicide.

A study published by Buiting *et al.* (2008) randomly selected a stratified sample of 2,100 physicians in the Netherlands and asked them about decision-making related to requests for euthanasia and assisted suicide. They found that 75% of the physicians who responded (56% response rate) had received such requests and 25% of the physicians who received requests had experienced problems in their decision-making with regard to at least one of the requirements for access to euthanasia and assisted suicide. Of the physicians who experienced problems, 79% had difficulties concerning the determination of whether or not the patient's suffering was unbearable and hopeless, and 58% had problems determining whether the request was voluntary or well considered. The same doubt about unbearable suffering criteria was reported by general practitioners who practised euthanasia (de Boer *et al.*, 2019). The authors of this study questioned whether the opinions of physicians, who often report difficulties in determining if the patients meet requirements for access to physician-assisted death, should be the basis of determining who should live or die according to the Dutch Euthanasia Act.

End-of-life decisions are also influenced by our fears and anxieties about the future – in this instance, our fears of dying. Research on fears about death has demonstrated that there is a panoply of common fears associated with the process of dying. The most common fears are of experiencing pain, losing control, dying alone, feeling humiliated or undignified, and being horribly incapacitated and dependent. Despite the fact that the majority of people have these concerns (Kastenbaum, 2000), research on the actual experience of the end of life indicates that these fears are generally unwarranted, especially when terminally ill people receive good hospice or palliative care (Hauswirth *et al.*, 2021; Kastenbaum, 2000).

For example, a study of patients suffering from ALS found that the most commonly reported reason for unbearable suffering in euthanasia requests in the Netherlands was fear of suffocation, accounting for 45% of requests (Maessen *et al.*, 2010). The same pattern was observed for ALS patients in states in the USA that have legalised assisted suicide (Hauswirth *et al.*, 2021). ALS patients actually have a very low incidence of suffocation in the terminal phase (0–3%), and there are available means for preventing this.

There is a remarkable discrepancy between what we know is right and best and human behaviour. Some smokers do not accept free programmes to stop smoking, even if they admit that it would be better for them. This ability to know what is best for oneself but still continue to do things that do not make us happier, healthier, or reduce our suffering has been called 'the neurotic paradox' (Shapiro, 1965). We may know that there is assistance to alleviate suffering, but that does not mean that we will necessarily seek it out. We admittedly have a tendency to make decisions based upon our fantasies and projections of future experiences, which may not accurately predict how we will react when the future arrives. For example, caregivers think that the majority of people with Alzheimer's disease would prefer to die rather than continue living with the illness, when in reality research has found that only between 3.2% (Draper *et al.*, 1998) and 14% (Holmstrand *et al.*, 2021) of Alzheimer's patients wished to die or had thoughts of death, and these sentiments fluctuate over time.

8.12   The Duty to Die: Contemporary Conceptions

Chapter 1 discussed in detail the contention that there may exist a duty to end one's life by suicide under certain circumstances. In that chapter we discussed how dying for a greater cause has occurred throughout history. It has been postulated that the change in the position of the Catholic

Church, from the early acceptance of altruistic suicides of martyrs to condemning suicide as sinful, may have been motivated by a concern that the most devout practitioners were dying too often by suicide (Murray, 2000). The classic sociological study by Durkheim (1985) described both egoistic and altruistic suicides, resulting from either marginalisation and alienation from society or over-identification and integration, as in the case of martyrs. Nowadays, concerns about choosing to die in order to benefit others are being expressed in the context of the choice to die by MAiD.

It appears that when individuals express their desire to end their lives by MAiD to avoid burdening others, this is accepted as a plausible motivation. However, if others exercise pressure on patients to die early to make their own life easier, this is regarded as unethical and therefore unacceptable. The Swiss government passed laws that stipulate that anyone may have access to assisted suicide, as long as there will be no personal gain for the person who assists. Whenever legalisation is debated, there is concern that euthanasia and assisted suicide not be practised in order to alleviate the financial burden on families or free up a hospital bed for an acute care patient in need of treatment.

People generally make sacrifices for others, ranging from trivial behaviours, such as sharing a larger portion of food, to heroic actions, as in risking one's life to protect family members. Laws and regulations about access to euthanasia and assisted suicide allow only for the reasons of personal pain and suffering. Nevertheless, human behaviour is often motivated by the need to please others and by concerns about meeting their needs. Sometimes those concerns may not be realistic. People who think that they are a burden to others often ignore the fact that caregivers can receive pleasure or satisfaction from taking care of a loved one. They may feel cheated of that opportunity when a person chooses to die prematurely by MAiD.

Religious concepts of duty to God may guide believers in end-of-life decisions. If one believes that only God may decide when and how a person will die, then euthanasia and assisted suicide are clearly forbidden. However, one may also have non-theological values of responsibility to family and community that can guide decision-making. These values can serve to motivate and justify MAiD, but may equally function to inhibit these practices. This inevitably depends upon the context. In some cultures, the concept of honour killing exists, to preserve cultural values. Consider the practice (now banned but still occasionally practised) in India of suttee, where the widow is expected to throw herself on the funeral pyre of her husband; if she refuses, family members may force her to do so. Another example is the suicide of a pregnant girl out of wedlock in Somaliland, who dies by suicide because of her desire to protect the honour of the family. There is the often-cited example, with questionable basis in fact, of the traditional Inuit elder who chooses to leave the village in winter for certain death when there is a scarcity of nourishment.

Altruistic euthanasia is rarely discussed, and its practice is excluded from legal requirements of who should have access to euthanasia and assisted suicide. On the other hand, social responsibilities and altruism may also be used to justify choosing to extend one's life despite suffering from a terminal or degenerative illness. There may be a wish to continue living to present a role model for others about how to confront death. Also, one might commit to stay alive to remain available to others as a community and family resource.

8.13 The Commodification of Life and the Customising of Death

Generally, in Western societies individual self-expression is increasing as we have greater opportunities to customise our life and lifestyle. Furthermore, in capitalist societies one may view one's life as a commodity whose value to oneself and to others may be greater or lesser, depending upon what pleasures we derive from life extension and how that contributes to others and to society as a whole. In a society where the value of objects, and of life itself, may be calculated, one may assess the worth of continuing to live in comparison to the worth of dying. Very often, people promoting a 'dignified' death speak of continuing to live in terms that suggest diminishing returns for the 'investment'. However, as in all material analyses, intangible and unanticipated factors may influence decision-making. Fear of death and dying, the inclination to stay with loved ones as long as possible, and similar factors may influence how we deal with the commodity of life.

Often it is the fear of anticipated suffering, rather than actual suffering itself, that leads people who are ill to end their lives. There has been considerable research attention to why cancer patients choose suicide, since they constitute by far the vast majority of those who have died by euthanasia and assisted suicide in countries where these practices have been legalised, including Canada, the Netherlands, Belgium, and the US states of Oregon and Washington. A review by Spoletini *et al.* (2011) and another by Robson *et al.* (2010) found that the risk of suicide in people with cancer is highest in the first year after diagnosis, especially in the first 3–5 months, but declines thereafter. This has been interpreted by the authors as reflecting the fact that patients who receive a diagnosis of cancer are forced to face a life-threatening experience, leading to painful emotions that may increase suicide risk. The periods immediately after receiving the diagnosis and following discharge from the hospital appear to be the times people are at highest risk of suicide (Calati *et al.*, 2021), because of the emotional impact of learning about the diagnosis and the difficult psychological adjustment outside of the hospital environment (Calati *et al.*, 2021; Lin *et al.*, 2009; Miccinesi *et al.*, 2004; Tanaka *et al.*, 1999). The authors also conclude that the risk is greatest if there is a psychiatric disorder present, as well as if the patient is experiencing physical pain. Following the period of initial shock and the beginning of treatment, usually after the first 3–5 months of living with the disease, the risk of suicide declines substantially.

There are a number of other significant risk factors for suicide in cancer patients, including having poor social support; loss of independence; fear of being a burden; having previously attempted suicide; being single, divorced, or widowed; and being male. However, the most powerful predictor of a desire for hastening death is major depression. In a study by Brown *et al.* (1986), all patients who reported the desire for rapid death (23% of the sample) were diagnosed with a major depression. Research indicates that cancer patient suicide is not just a reaction to the diagnosis and to suffering from the disease, but it is also associated with psychological vulnerability to stress, which may be caused or exacerbated by immunological disturbances that often occur when people have cancer. The hypothesis that immunological disturbances may weaken one's ability to deal with stress is controversial and needs better substantiation in research.

8.14   End-of-Life Practices in an Ideal Universe

Countries differ greatly in the extent and nature of their intrusions into the lives of their citizens. There are major differences in the control of lifestyles and the availability of social benefits. The Netherlands, the first country to accept the practice and legalise euthanasia and assisted suicide, is liberal in terms of its respect for individual freedom. It was one of the first countries to allow for marijuana to be legally purchased, and prostitution is legal. However, the Netherlands also provides universal health care for its citizens and has a fairly extensive network of palliative care. The *Economist* ranked the Netherlands as seventh in overall quality of end-of-life care and Belgium fifth, in comparison with 40 other countries (Economist Intelligence Unit, 2010). These countries are part of a wide spectrum of other sociopolitical systems that exist in the world, ranging from ultra-liberal constitutional structures to dictatorial monarchies and theocratic regimes. It is highly relevant to analyse the legalisation of euthanasia and assisted suicide in the context of the nature of government, the culture of individualism, and the availability of alternatives to ending life.

In a theocratic country, end-of-life decisions are determined by religious prescripts and there is little room for promoting individual freedoms that may go against fundamental beliefs. This model of a paternalistic society is one of many ways that a country may regulate practices in what it considers the best interest of its citizens.

A society with a communitarian ethos may continually strive to do what is best for the masses, to the detriment of individual choice. Where the state works to protect its citizens, how should one assess the value to citizens of making euthanasia and assisted suicide available? Where there are limited resources for health care, it may be for the greater good to have unproductive, ill people who drain valuable resources end their lives as early as possible in order to ensure that resources are equitably distributed. From another perspective, does respect for individual rights imply not only respect for the manner of dying, but an obligation on the part of the state to provide the means (assisted suicide) and the manpower (in the case of euthanasia) to end life on demand?

Few liberal democratic societies are homogeneous in terms of religious beliefs and values. How should these issues be legislated in a pluralistic, multicultural society with a range of affinities? A common response is that permitting MAiD does not obligate any person to choose that option. However, expectations can play a large part in medical practice. At the beginning of the twentieth century, it was considered to be 'normal' and ethical for women to suffer during childbirth. Now, it is generally considered unethical to not offer help to control women's pain.

In the Netherlands, a study (Onwuteaka-Philipsen *et al.*, 2012) reported that two thirds of requests for euthanasia did not lead to euthanasia or physician-assisted suicide being performed. In about half the instances where the person's request for euthanasia was not carried out, the person had died before the request was granted. In one third of people who requested euthanasia, the physician denied the request because it was felt that the request was not well considered and/or the patient was found to not be suffering unbearably. In the opinion of the physicians, due-care criteria obligated them to not grant euthanasia since the patient had not exhausted other means of dealing with the problems that had resulted in their requesting physician-assisted death by euthanasia. When the physician denied the request for euthanasia, indicating that other treatments or help should be tried first, patients rarely returned with their request. These data suggest that in a substantial number of cases, even in a country where euthanasia is a well-established practice supported by a majority of the population and the medical community, when patients tell doctors that they have insupportable suffering or loss of dignity, this is not necessarily well-founded and the problems are not really insurmountable.

8.15 A Thought Experiment: A Society with 'Ideal' End-of-Life Practises?

For some, the ideal situation for end-of-life care would be a society where all citizens enjoy the optimum medical and psychosocial treatment and palliative care at home is provided to meet all the terminally ill person's needs. This benevolent social state would also provide all the needed support for the family of the dying person, including respite care at a hospice if the family needs to take a regular or periodic break from being involved in caregiving. This was the dream of Dr Cecily Saunders when she founded the hospice movement in England (Richmond, 2005). It was her contention that if a full range of good palliative care is provided to terminally ill people and their families, there would be no need to debate the legalisation of euthanasia or assisted suicide. No one would experience the physical and psychological suffering that could motivate people to want to end their life prematurely. A Cochrane Review of research on hospice care at home (Gomes *et al.*, 2013) concluded that there is 'clear and reliable evidence' that home palliative care reduces 'symptom burden'. A more recent systematic review has confirmed this conclusion (Zimbroff *et al.*, 2021).

For the late Supreme Court judge of the Netherlands Huib Drion, the ideal society in terms of end-of-life care would provide all citizens when they reached maturity (probably at age 18) with a pill with which they could end their life at any time, if they felt that it would be unbearable to continue living (Drion, 1992). For Drion, the exercise of the decision to live or die is an inalienable right in a free and just society, and that right should be able to be exercised without any meddling by governments. He felt that knowing that we can die whenever we choose would provide a sense of freedom to live life fully, and would provide for the utmost fulfilment in everyone's life.

This example can be both supported and criticised on philosophical and practical grounds. The example of the society where every aspect of end-of-life care is provided to ensure that all needs are met follows from a view of society as having extensive responsibilities to ensure that all citizens are provided the very best of care. Some may contend that such a maternalistic society would be stifling of individual freedom. Others doubt that all people suffering from illnesses can have their suffering reduced, or that being dependent upon caregivers is not a dignified way to live or die. One may question if the benefits are justified by the costs involved, feeling that the money could be better spent helping others who are not so ill.

Drion's (1992) utopia of each person deciding when to die can be criticised as overemphasising individual freedom at the expense of people's obligations to loved ones and society at large. Critics predict dire consequences of having death so easily available, as people may carelessly kill themselves while inebriated or in a temporary crisis situation.

Between these two extreme views of the role of the state and individual freedom to choose to die, one may envision a wide range of alternative models. Globally, we live in an imperfect world where people have false beliefs, unsubstantiated fears, biases, and prejudices; where they sometimes kill or want to exterminate others for tribal reasons; where there are intergenerational conflicts about sharing of resources; and where obligations are not always respected. Medical personnel are burdened with time and resource constraints and may have human prejudices.

Despite the possibility of holding an extreme position favouring an absolute right of individuals to choose to die when and how they please in industrial democracies, citizens continue to live in places where governments are increasingly enacting legislation to protect their citizens from engaging in behaviours that compromise their health and well-being. Sometimes the motivations for these actions may appear to be based on benefits for the state, despite their obvious benefits for the population. For example, one of the motivations for anti-smoking regulations is the reduction of health-care expenses for treating smoking-related illness. In the case of MAiD, if one puts the moral arguments aside, in many instances there is a delicate balance between corporate interests of the state and the benefits to citizens.

In many modern societies where there is a secular government that purports to be neutral with regard to religious morality, the lack of absolute moral principles leads to more practical discussions, with the underlying moral principles being implicit and hidden behind practical concerns. Under these circumstances, we tend to use consequentialist arguments about the benefits for the 'individual' of having access to different practices and the risks involved. It is taken for granted that there are no moral imperatives that would contravene what is proposed.

Very little of the current debates examines perceived and morally explained obligations to family and society. Chapter 1 presented the philosophical arguments for a duty to die, as well as arguments for an obligation to intervene to protect life. There is sometimes a thin line between the desire to die earlier for the sake of others and the choice of a premature death as a result of pressure to free up a bed needed for other patients, or family concerns about the high cost of care. It is important, to the extent possible, for individuals who must decide whether or not to approve a request for MAiD to be keenly aware of these potential pressures.

8.16 Conclusions

The main issue in the debate over the legalisation of MAiD is the balance between respect for autonomous freedom of choice and the obligations of the state to protect citizens against their potentially distorted or unrealistic beliefs. Hitherto there has been a tendency to err more towards protecting life rather than respecting freedom of choice. The obligation in the Netherlands is to alleviate suffering before allowing access to euthanasia or assisted suicide. That all other means must first be tried constitutes a moral middle ground between respecting individual freedom to choose to die and protecting citizens from making an irrevocable decision based upon the false premise that their suffering will be interminable.

In Canada, the obligation to alleviate suffering before having access to death as the solution (i.e., MAiD) has been replaced by the obligation of physicians to inform patients of other potential means for alleviating their suffering (Mishara and Kerkhof, 2018). However, the physician cannot refuse access to MAiD to a person who decides not to try the treatments the doctor believes will diminish the person's suffering without resorting to ending the person's life. In Canada, if the patient does not feel that the proposed treatment is 'acceptable', the physician is obligated to provide death by MAiD. The lack of a requirement in Canada to withhold death to end suffering when the physician thinks there are other options may explain why in 2021 more people died by MAiD in Canada than in any other country.

We cannot help wondering how much of the current desire to allow and support people in choosing how and when to die is a continuation of an age-old attempt to assuage our fears that we all risk dying at a time that we do not decide and in a manner that we cannot control. We live in an age where suffering is not valued, where we take medication to make us feel better when we are grieving, where we seek to control all pain, and imagine that any psychological angst can be reversed by a good therapist. In this context it is no wonder that the prospect of dying and the anticipatory anxiety that the process of being terminally ill or incapacitated evokes can be viewed as antithetical to all we have been trying to attain in our lives. If we believe that death cannot be controlled or avoided, then the only options that remain in order to maintain psychological calm is to either accept a dying process that we can little control, while receiving palliative care for the pain and emotional suffering, or to die by MAiD. By choosing MAiD we may assert our autonomous personhood by cheating death of its haphazard destruction of the self. Finally, we should contemplate that if the desire to have governments facilitate our access to an earlier death by MAiD is related to our fear-based expectations of the dying process, then, besides debating the legal, moral, and practical concerns, we should also focus upon the psychological roots of our fears and examine ways to reduce those fears in individuals and societies.

9

· · · · · · ·

Suicide Prevention and the Expansion of Medical Assistance in Dying

9.1 Introduction

Suicide prevention services do their utmost to prevent suicides with all people, regardless of the suicidal individual's characteristics and the reasons given for wanting to die. The assumption is that doing otherwise constitutes discrimination and that it would create an ethical morass to attempt to determine whether some lives are more worthy of saving than others. Doctors are meant to work equally hard to save the life of a wounded murderer as they do with the victim of a homicide attempt. The suicidal 90-year-old patient who has cancer should obtain the same quality of suicide prevention services as the teenager who was abandoned by a significant other. In the context where MAiD is available, should we continue to strive to prevent all suicides, or are there some circumstances where we should abstain from preventing a death by suicide, or even encourage people to seek MAiD?

9.2   Suicide Prevention in Theory and in Practice

We live in a post-Kantian universe, with many societies dominated by the paradigms of secular humanism and modern-day versions of relativism. We tend increasingly to reject religious dogma and absolutes as the basis of morality and decision-making. Moralists who persist in claiming that suicide prevention is an absolute moral obligation have been pressured to concede that there might be exceptions that should be considered.

There are competing interests that have to be considered, depending on the context. Some have described the current ethical state of affairs by using the philosophical vocabulary of quasi-absolutes, which on the face of it sounds like a contradiction. Exceptions indeed are exceptions, and, in the matter of suicide, because death is absolute and irreversible, great care must be taken to find a connection between our competing values and the outcomes that we deem necessary to maintain an acceptable level of either social or individual conscience.

In most situations, people working in suicide prevention are comfortable with the policies of their mandate to prevent suicide without differentiation based on personal characteristics or the reasons people give to decide to end their lives. Nevertheless, it is a reasonable assumption that distinctions are sometimes made. Decisions are in the hands of individual practitioners, who may be influenced by their emotional reactions or resource scarcity considerations, even when those reactions are in conflict with official policies. Such compromises in practices that may go against stated policies bring into question the moral judgement of those responsible to protect the vulnerable. The practical reality is, whether it is the absolute value of human life that is the ultimate reference or the fact that people, after they have been prevented from attempting suicide, are more often than not thankful, there remains a matter of conscience about what to do when there is an articulated assertion in favour of or against ending or assisting in ending anyone's life. In jurisdictions where MAiD is legal, there is no interference with the desire to hasten death, and direct interventions to terminate life are available in some specified circumstances.

In practice, suicide prevention workers may face moral dilemmas in conforming to the mandate of helping everyone despite the circumstances. In a silent monitoring study, where Mishara *et al.* (2007) listened to 2,611 calls to United States helplines, there were a very small number of calls (four) where helpers actually encouraged the caller to proceed with their suicide attempt. These were extreme situations. For example, one caller, standing on a bridge, told how he was unsuccessful in desisting from raping his 6-year-old daughter and, since he was unable to arrest this practice through therapy, he had decided to end his life. After having explored all the treatments and options and after deciding that the person was in fact incorrigible, the helpline worker expressed the view that it was acceptable to jump. Although this went against the ethical standards of the helpline, it does point out the common-sense observation that even in the suicide prevention universe there can be an outlook, prejudicial or not, that there are people deserving of death.

9.3   The Advent of Medical Assistance in Dying

After decades of volatile debate, the international trend is to create exceptions to the historically stated absolute mandate to prevent death (see Chapter 8). We are witnessing a push towards the legalisation of MAiD. The legal provision of death for some people has opened up a public dialogue about identifying categories of people or motives for wanting to die. This conversation leads away from having a firm and limited set of criteria towards a spirit of progressive liberalism in expanding access to MAiD. There are heated debates where well-honed arguments about obligations to protect vulnerable populations are presented (e.g., Cohen-Almagor, 2009; Lerner & Caplan, 2015; see Chapter 8 of this book).

9.4 Are There Justified Distinctions Between How to Respond to People Requesting MAiD and Suicidal Individuals?

In earlier decades, when the legalisation of MAiD ('euthanasia' and 'assisted suicide) was first openly discussed, the dangers of the 'slippery slope' were widely recognised. It was feared that once the door was open, MAiD would be expanded and made available to people who were not experiencing the original criteria of intolerable suffering from an irreversible terminal illness. This concern is much less evident in contemporary debates.

An autonomy-based mantra now dominates the discourse in Western countries. Nevertheless, there is a critical literature that is tantamount to the slippery-slope critique, where authors have expressed serious trepidation about misguided applications, their perception being that MAiD risks the miscarriage of justice. As described in detail in previous chapters, in Switzerland, Belgium, the Netherlands and Canada, MAiD, which was initially available only to people who were already dying or at an advanced stage of a severe degenerative physical illness, is now available to people whose suffering is solely from mental health problems (or is planned to be available in 2024 in Canada).

The Netherlands was the pioneer in MAiD legislation. It was the first country to eliminate criminal euthanasia and assisted suicide by judicial decisions, beginning in 1973, and was the first to pass legislation to eliminate punishment for physicians who engage in practices to terminate life if their due-care criteria were followed. They were to first to allow MAiD for people whose suffering was only attributed to a mental illness.

In the Netherlands, in 2016, Pi Dijkstra, a member of the Second Chamber of the Parliament, presented a proposal to allow euthanasia and assisted suicide for 'a completed life' for any person who is over age 75 and tired of living, without any requirement that the person must have a mental or physical condition as a cause, or that intolerable suffering must be a part of the request (D66, 2016). Dijkstra argued that more mature elders are better able to assess the future quality of their remaining life, old age is a period when there is increasing likelihood of being lonely and physically dependent, and fixing an age threshold would be a source of peace and reassurance by setting a goal to live towards.

In reaction to the proposal, Paul Schnabel, a First Chamber member representing the same D66 political party, in a report from the legislative advice committee that studied the legislative proposition, agreed with the law, but said the age limitation was arbitrary and should be eliminated, since everyone ages at their own pace and it is only the feelings experienced that matter (Schnabel *et al.*, 2016). The committee felt that setting an age threshold would be stigmatising to the elderly, and they recommended that the law should be passed, allowing euthanasia for people any of age who are tired of living.

The proposal would change the current requirement that requests to terminate life be vetted by two doctors, to establish a new type of professional, an 'end-of-life coordinator', who would have ethical and medical training, would receive and assess the request, and would be able to perform the euthanasia safely and comfortably. The proposal stipulated that the end-of-life coordinator would receive special training on how to relate appropriately to existential questions concerning detachment, loss of identity, and loss of purpose (D66, 2016). The practice of ending life under this legislation was described as an assisted suicide.

The end-of-life coordinator would have three principal responsibilities: to establish that the request is without external pressure, to establish that the decision is well considered and durable, and to prescribe medication to the requester and remain present when the lethal medication is taken. Unlike physicians, whose primary role is to heal and who can provide euthanasia or assisted suicide only if they determine that interventions to diminish the patient's mental and physical suffering are not possible, the only role of the end-of-life coordinator would be to decide whether to end the person's life.

The D66 party, which backed the proposal, was divided over the issue of setting an age threshold for allowing euthanasia and assisted suicide versus allowing termination of life for everyone who is tired of living. Holzman (2021) contended that in principle, euthanasia on the basis of a completed life could be morally permissible, but there are serious moral implementation problems in the proposal because of the potential for ageist stigma if an age threshold is set, and it will be difficult to determine if the decision is truly well considered and durable if people of any age can terminate life only because they are tired of living. Holzman (2021) has recognised that requiring physicians to end the lives of individuals who are not ill could be ethically unacceptable, and questioned the emotional ability of end-of-life coordinators to fulfil their requisite duties.

In 2022, the Council of State, a constitutionally established advisory body to the government and Parliament, determined that the proposal should not be adopted, since it contains insufficient safety guarantees. The Council cited research showing that, in some cases, the desire to die diminishes or disappears over time. They contended that the desire might be related to medical problems or problems that could be resolved. Although the Council's recommendation is non-binding, and the proposal could still be voted upon, as of March 2023, no vote was taken.

If this legislation were eventually to pass, what would distinguish a suicidal person whose life we should try to save from a person tired of living and who is exercising the right to choose death without experiencing suffering? If having a mental illness that influences the ability to reason and a clinical depression obscuring hope for future improvement were included as an exclusion criterion, this would eliminate about 90% of suicidal individuals in high-income countries. However, the Netherlands does not exclude people with mental illness from accessing euthanasia and assisted suicide.

If the age threshold of 75 is retained in the proposal, suicide prevention organisations could limit their interventions to younger people. However, they could maintain their provision of help to everyone, including people tired of living who want to explore the possibility of regaining hope by contacting suicide prevention organisations. If the legislation is adopted, it remains to be seen how this could affect emergency treatment and hospitalisation of suicidal individuals and people who attempt suicide (see Chapter 8). We wonder whether, if this legislative proposal is adopted in the Netherlands, other countries will again eventually follow in their footsteps.

9.5 Is There a Difference Between MAiD and Suicide?

Several organisations have proposed that there is a clear distinction between suicide and MAiD. The American Association of Suicidology (2017) had stated that there are fifteen ways in which suicide and MAiD differ. As the basis for their proposed distinctions, they took the nature of MAiD as it is practised in some states of the USA, where assisted suicide has been legalised only for people who are terminally ill. Their distinctions described how the practice and implications of MAiD differ from the practice of ending one's life. For example, they noted that with MAiD, the patient is mainly surrounded by family at the time of death, whereas suicides normally occur in isolation. In fact, it is illegal for others to be present and thus encourage, help, or assist a person to end their life in most countries, including all countries where MAiD is permitted (see Chapter 7). Another distinction pointed to the 'interminable suffering' component in MAiD. Suicide was considered to be a way of coping with suffering that is perceived to be interminable and omnipresent. Despite the aforementioned range of distinctions that describe the respective nature of the practices of MAiD and suicide, there are in fact no viable research findings to date that indicate that one can reliably distinguish between people who are appropriate candidates for MAiD and suicidal individuals who would benefit from suicide prevention interventions. The American Association of Suicidology has since rescinded this contention that there is a distinction between suicide and physician aid in dying and has removed the text describing the alleged distinctions from their website.

If the experience of great suffering does not allow us to successfully distinguish between people who die by suicide and people who seek or receive MAiD, is there another avenue to distinguish them? If MAiD is limited to people who are already dying, or where death is foreseeable, then it can be argued that MAiD is truly distinguishable from suicide, based on the fact that in MAiD, people choose to alter the manner and timing of a foreseeable death, while in the case of suicide, a person chooses to die when death is not already going to occur in the near future.

We might theoretically postulate that there is less ambivalence about changing the manner and timing of death when a terminally ill person requests MAiD, compared with ending the life of a physically healthy person. However, as we have emphasised in Chapters 1 and 8, the reality is that people seeking medically assisted death are not consistently making clear choices without ambivalence, as happens with most human decisions. There are a host of influences that confuse the decision-making process. For example, side effects of medications used to treat physical illnesses are often accompanied by depression and its associated feelings of hopelessness (e.g., chemotherapy for cancer, Parkinson's disease medications). In the absence of empirical data that allow us to determine when the desire to die by MAiD can or cannot be alleviated, we may contend that there is a moral imperative to always provide help and intervene before a request to die by MAiD is granted.

Feelings of hopelessness are seminal to suicide and MAiD choices. In the case of MAiD, it is assumed that the feeling of hopelessness reflects the reality of the circumstances: There is no way of relieving the person's suffering. When that suffering is associated with the imminence of death and the symptoms of an incapacitating terminal illness, the lack of hope is generally justified by the lack of a cure for the illness, assuming that the suffering is an inevitable consequence of the medical condition and its effects. However, people who work in hospices and in palliative care contend that in most cases, the suffering of terminally ill people can be alleviated or substantially diminished, so that the desire to die prematurely is averted (Richmond, 2005). Similarly, the ethos of suicide prevention is in its essence connected to the goal of diminishing hopelessness and embracing the possibility of regaining a desire for sustaining life. In the absence of empirical data that reliably indicate who can and cannot regain the will to continue living, providing help is the only way to determine whether hope can be increased and the desire to die can be significantly diminished.

9.6   Suicide Prevention and the Liberal Zeitgeist

Without reliable criteria to distinguish between suicides and MAiD requests, what are the parameters for suicide prevention that can be guidelines for best practice? Should suicide prevention groups maintain their policies to always intervene, owing to the overriding value of saving lives whenever possible? Where should suicide prevention policymakers draw the limits of intervention in a manner helpful in their day-to-day practice? Given the lack of empirical evidence on the critical issue of the range and types of ambivalence that occur in real-life situations in MAiD, it is probable that suicide prevention groups will continue to maintain their policy of offering interventions in almost every case, owing to the belief that saving lives, despite recent trends, is a mandate that has stood the test of time.

In the past, Thomas Szasz (1986) argued that suicide prevention activities should be abandoned in favour of an absolute respect for individual autonomy. His arguments have been generally ignored by the suicide prevention community, based on its belief that respecting autonomy does not preclude offering and actively providing help to suicidal individuals. Also, people involved in suicide prevention contend that the ability to make autonomous decisions without undue influence is often already compromised.

To deprive people who meet the criteria for MAiD of the opportunity to receive suicide prevention interventions by putting them in a category apart has no empirical or clinically reliable justification. Providing help to all without discrimination is not incompatible with respect for autonomous decision-making. Offering suicide prevention interventions to all provides an opportunity for some people who otherwise would have died prematurely to regain the will to live, regardless of their circumstances.

10

• • • • • • •

Conclusion: My Brother's Keeper

In this book, we explored three core positions that dominate the current spectrum of applied ethics in suicide prevention. Our perspective is that while there are areas of consensus statements among professional groups, institutions, and in the academic literature, there are distinct orientations that have historical precedents and associations with characteristic social attitudes, albeit with inevitable overlaps and confusing internal contradictions. This book delineated three ethical perspectives: moralist, libertarian, and relativist.

The moralists, who contend that suicide is always unacceptable and must be prevented, have occupied the mainstream position through a long period of history. Moralist roots can be found in the Greco-Roman rejection of taking one's life except in the context of a sacrifice for a higher purpose, such as the celebrity cases of Socrates, Thrasea Paetus, and Cato Uticensis. Saint Augustine and Thomas Aquinas later set aside the tradition of an honourable aristocrat sacrificing life in the name of a higher social purpose, or a Christian martyr dying for his beliefs, with the introduction of Christian views about suicide as being an affront to the Divine, who alone can give and take away life. That view, shared in Muslim and Jewish teachings, persisted for centuries. Following the very public display of violation of the body of the person who died by suicide, families of the suicide perpetrator were punished with warning signals to the community by the usurpation of family property by churches and rulers.

This punitive reaction to suicide continued for many centuries until superseded by modifications that arrived in Europe with the Enlightenment, when people turned towards science. The problem of suicide was medicalised as a species of insanity, to be treated by strict forms of medical paternalism. The asylums created by the Church and by secular institutions, which continued into the early twentieth century, viewed suicidal individuals with demeaning attitudes as people who were dangerous and deviant.

Attacks on the moralistic point of view were highlighted in the twentieth century by the writings of such anti-psychiatrists as Szasz (1986), who argued that all suicide prevention should be abandoned, and thereafter by more philosophical critics such as Foucault (1976). Critiques of paternalistic incarceration resulted in emancipatory movements away from the asylum and towards heightening the virtue of freedom and the right to choose one's treatment. This movement, broadly called *libertarianism*, worked its way through the latter part of the twentieth century and into the twenty-first, attempting to free mental disorders from stigmatisation and eliminating the second-order citizenship of women and many minority groups. Some have allied with 'autonomists', who advocate that admittedly mentally disordered people have the right to avoid even well-meaning interventions by suicide prevention groups, and support those who, because of incurable and unacceptable suffering of a mental nature, choose to end their lives independently or with assistance.

Because of the great numbers who identify as libertarians, even people working in so-called progressive suicide prevention groups (e.g., American Association of Suicidology, 2017) have retreated into positions of accommodation best described as within the spectrum of ethical relativism. The predicament we face in the early twenty-first century is whether these accommodations reveal a disassociation from concern for the vulnerable or whether we as a society believe that the choice to suicide is beyond the judgement of fellow citizens. Since the age of extreme moralism, suicide has retreated into a dramatically changed environment of the 'private' superseding the 'public', so much so that the principles of the ancients and philosophers of the Enlightenment may now appear to be essentially inapplicable to modern concerns and even to ethical instincts.

There are certain ironies that present themselves in this century. For example, in such ultraconservative theocratic societies as Iran, we find very well-organised suicide prevention groups, despite the Muslim tradition that considers suicide attempts sinful behaviour. Why is this so? Perhaps because there has been a creeping acceptance, even in traditional Abrahamic religious communities, of the potential for sinful acts to be averted. If a suicide attempt can be prevented by religious care, by chaplaincy, and through benevolent acts or psychiatric interventions, this religiously sanctioned behaviour can be prevented, and the contravening of severe religious interventions effectively averted.

On the libertarian side, other ironies are present. The legislative proposal in the hands of the legislature of the Netherlands proposes that people over a certain age, even if in good mental and physical health, should be able to choose euthanasia or assisted suicide without any reason other than their conclusion that ongoing life is no longer 'worth living'. How is it possible that liberal and highly tolerant secular democracies have step-by-step advanced in favour of facilitating the ending of life, and in some very theocratic societies there are increasing interventions to preserve life?

How have these existential imbalances been created, and what can we foresee for the future in terms of trends and policies? What is the true substance of tolerance that appears to result in a dissociative morality where individualism of the extreme libertarian sort is accepted essentially without comment, critique, or judgement? Have we moved away from a caring morality in the twenty-first century, as a reaction to the many political, social, and even moral revolutions? Has this happened because we hold a view in the developed economies that civilisation has abandoned collective moral responsibility, so we cling to an extreme individualism?

During the COVID-19 pandemic, we have observed increasing numbers of educated people in so-called liberal democracies who are resistant to the idea of social responsibility in vaccination policies, isolation rules, and wearing masks. Adding to that is a plethora of support for autocratic regimes and cults of leadership.

Michel Foucault (1976) has described an amalgamation of structures in professional groups, economies, and governing instruments of power that consider those wanting to die by suicide as 'the other', seen through the authoritarian glance of one holding power against a disenfranchised group who are held down – in fact, enslaved – through a brainwashing of low esteem and denial of self. The only way out of such a miserable condition is through a rethinking of identity and self.

How can we translate these insights into practical outcomes that are beneficial and go beyond the realm of philosophical insight? If we do not want to surrender to the 'autonomists' because we fear a culture of abandonment, can we address the relativism of the twenty-first century by claiming some core values? Searching for middle ground should not amount to a series of compromises, but must involve a clear direction of 'centrepiece values' that allow for the continuance of respectful suicide prevention policies.

In a recent book, *Ontologie du devenir*, the renowned public intellectual Anne Fagot-Largeault (Fagot-Largeault *et al.*, 2021) proclaimed that the ancient philosopher Heraclitus remains the most perceptive of all philosophers to have discovered that life and its values are in an endless state of becoming, and that 'being', the grand go-to ontological reality of philosophy and history, even in the world of astrophysics and the awareness of ever-expanding galaxies, has underscored the Heraclitan statement of all things changing, a never-ending dialectic of transformation. This way of looking, of perceiving the state of values, is expressed in the great texts of Hegel, Nietzsche, Wittgenstein, and the controversial texts of the ethical relativists that followed the positivists into the controversies of the twenty-first century.

We have observed religious institutions decomposing and political activism so extreme that if there is a need in the twenty-first century, it is to find what still creates a consensus, a basis, or 'civicalisation' for the rediscovery of something in the consciousness of civilisation that is ecologically and humanistically sensitive. Can we not learn from climate change and our inhumane treatment of others, that without a caring philosophy of rescue, there is a decreasing quantum of morality in Western consciousness?

Suicide prevention should be seen as a central issue that has to be assessed alongside the anti-paternalism promotion of freedom of choice. The concern of this book has not been to find a middle ground. We have sought a social and moral conscience that mandates a duty to respond to suicide and the desire to end life prematurely, first and foremost, by responding to cries for help, rather than to a clarion call for freedom.

References

Penal Code (Northern States) Federal Provisions Act. *No. 25 of 1960*.

1943. Lebanon penal code. Lebanon.

1962. Penal code. *5*. Somalia.

1984. Calder v. Jones. U.S. Supreme Court.

1993. Criminal code 1974. In Independent state of Papua New Guinea, *311*. Papua New Guinea.

1999. Braintech, Inc. v. Kostiuk. Court of appeal for British Columbia.

2001. R (Pretty) v Director of Public Prosecutions. United Kingdom House of Lords.

2002. R (Pretty) v United Kingdom. European Court of Human Rights.

2003. Act of Ghana. *29*. Ghana: First Republic of Ghana.

2004. Law No. 11 of 2004 Issuing the Penal Code. *11*. Qatar.

2006. Laws of Malaysia. *574*. Malaysia: The Commissioner of Law revision.

2008. The penal code act. *Chapter XVI*. South Sudan.

2009. R (On the application of Purdy) v Director of Public Prosecutions House of Lords.

2015. Penal code. *L.R.O. 1/2015* Malawi.

2016. Laws of Brunei. *Chapter 22 penal code*. Brunei: Attorney general's chamber.

2019. Penal Code. *Chapter XXII*. United Republic Tanzania.

2020. Criminal offence bill. *XXI*. Gambia.

[2012]. Rabone and another (Appellants) v Pennine Care NHS Trust (Respondent). *500–17–099119–177*. The Supreme Court.

[2016]. Daniel v St George's Healthcare NHS Trust and London Ambulance Service. England and Wales High Court.

[2019]-a. Olewnik-Cieplińska and Olewnik v. Poland. European Court of Human Rights (First Section).

[2019]-b. Truchon v. Attorney General of Canada and Attorney General of Québec. *500–17–099119–177*. Superior Court.

AHERN, S., BURKE, L. A., MCELROY, B., CORCORAN, P., MCMAHON, E. M., KEELEY, H., CARLI, V., WASSERMAN, C., HOVEN, C. W., SARCHIAPONE, M., APTER, A., BALAZS, J., BANZER, R., BOBES, J., BRUNNER, R., COSMAN, D., HARING, C., KAESS, M., KAHN, J. P., KERESZTENY, A., POSTUVAN, V.,

SÁIZ, P. A., VARNIK, P. & WASSERMAN, D. 2018. A cost-effectiveness analysis of school-based suicide prevention programmes. *European Child and Adolescent Psychiatry*, 27, 1295–1304.

ALACREU-CRESPO, A., CAZALS, A., COURTET, P. & OLIÉ, E. 2020. Brief assessment of psychological pain to predict suicidal events at one year in depressed patients. *Psychotherapy and Psychosomatics*, 89, 320–323.

ALAO, A. O., SODERBERG, M., POHL, E. L. & ALAO, A. L. 2006. Cybersuicide: review of the role of the internet on suicide. *CyberPsychology & Behavior*, 9, 489–493.

ALLEN, N. 2013. The right to life in a suicidal state. *International Journal of Law and Psychiatry*, 36, 350–357.

ALTMAN, M. C. 2020. Can suicide preserve one's dignity? Kant and Kantians on the moral response to cognitive loss. *Kant-Studien*, 111, 593–611.

AMERICAN ASSOCIATION OF SUICIDOLOGY 2017. *Statement of the American Association of Suicidology: Suicide is not the Same as Physician Aid in Dying.* Washington, DC: American Association of Suicidology.

ANDRIESSEN, K., REIFELS, L., KRYSINSKA, K., ROBINSON, J., DEMPSTER, G. & PIRKIS, J. 2019. Ethical concerns in suicide research: results of an international researcher survey. *Journal of Empirical Research on Human Research Ethics*, 14, 383–394.

ANGERS, A., KAGKLI, D. M., KOELLINGER, P., PETRILLO, M., QUERCI, M., RAFFAEL, B. & VAN DEN EDEE, G. 2019. *Genome-wide Association Studies, Polygenic Scores and Social Science Genetics: Overview and Policy Implications.* Luxembourg: Publications Office of the European Union.

ANGUS REID INSTITUTE 2023. Mental health and MAID: Canadians question looming changes to Canada's assisted-death law. https://angusreid.org/wp-content/uploads/2023/02/2023.02.13_MAID.pdf

APKARIAN, A. V., SOSA, Y., KRAUSS, B. R., THOMAS, P. S., FREDRICKSON, B. E., LEVY, R. E., HARDEN, R. N. & CHIALVO, D. R. 2004. Chronic pain patients are impaired on an emotional decision-making task. *Pain*, 108, 129–136.

APPELBAUM, P. S. 1994. *Almost a Revolution: Mental Health Law and the Limits of Change.* New York: Oxford University Press.

APPELBAUM, P. S. 2001. Thinking carefully about outpatient commitment. *Psychiatric Services*, 52, 347–350.

ARBOLEDA-FLÓREZ, J. & WEISSTUB, D. N. 2008. Mental health rights: the relation between constitution and bioethics. In WEISSTUB, D. N. & PINTOS,

G. D. (eds.) *Autonomy and Human Rights in Health Care: An International Perspective*. Dordrecht: Springer Netherlands.

ARISTOTLE 2000. *Nicomachean Ethics. Book I*. Alex Catalogue (Original work published BCE).

ARSENAULT-LAPIERRE, G., KIM, C. & TURECKI, G. 2004. Psychiatric diagnoses in 3275 suicides: a meta-analysis. *BMC Psychiatry*, 4, 37.

ASSEMBLÉE NATIONALE 2014. *Bill 52, An Act Respecting End-of-life Care. BILL 52*. Québec: Assemblée Nationale.

AUSTRALIAN IT. 2004. *Crackdown on suicide chat rooms*. [Online]. Available at: http://australianit.news.com.au/wireless/story/0,8256,10340811,00.html.

BACH, M. & KERZNER, L. 2010. *A New Paradigm for Protecting Autonomy and the Right to Legal Capacity*. Toronto: Law Commission of Ontario.

BAECHLER, J. (ed.) 1975. *Les suicides*. Berlin: Calmann-Lévy.

BAEVA, L. V. 2020. Social and existential threats to personal security in virtual communities: 'Groups of death' and 'Columbine communities'. *International Journal of Technoethics*, 11, 1–16.

BAGHRAMIAN, M. & CARTER, J. A. 2022. Relativism. In ZALTA, E. N. (ed.). *The Stanford Encyclopedia of Philosophy*. https://plato.stanford.edu/archives/spr2022/entries/relativism.

BAGNASCO, A., ZANINI, M., DASSO, N., ROSSI, S., TIMMINS, F., GALANTI, M. C., ALEO, G., CATANIA, G. & SASSO, L. 2020. *Dignity, Privacy, Respect and Choice: A Scoping Review of Measurement of These Concepts Within Acute Healthcare Practice*. Chichester: Wiley-Blackwell.

BAKER, E. A., BREWER, S. K., OWENS, J. S., COOK, C. R. & LYON, A. R. 2021. Dissemination science in school mental health: a framework for future research. *School Mental Health: A Multidisciplinary Research and Practice Journal*, 13, 791–807.

BARHAM, P. 1997. *Closing the Asylum: The Mental Patient in Modern Society*. London: Penguin.

BARRETT, D. H., ORTMANN, L. W. & LARSON, S. A. 2022. *Narrative Ethics in Public Health: The Value of Stories*. Cham: Springer.

BARROIS, G. A. 1945. *Basic Writings of Saint Thomas Aquinas*. New York: Random House.

BARTLETT, P. 2003. The test of compulsion in mental health law: capacity, therapeutic benefit and dangerousness as possible criteria. *Medical Law Review*, 11, 326–352.

BATTIN, M. P. 1984. The concept of rational suicide. In SHNEIDMAN, E. S. (ed.) *Death: Current Perspectives*. Palo Alto: Mayfield Publishing.

BAUME, P., CANTOR, C. H. & ROLFE, A. 1997. Cybersuicide: the role of interactive suicide notes on the internet. *Crisis: The Journal of Crisis Intervention and Suicide Prevention*, 18, 73–79.

BEAUCHAMP, T. L. & CHILDRESS, J. F. 2009. *Principles of Biomedical Ethics*. New York: Oxford University Press.

BECKER, K. & SCHMIDT, M. H. 2004. Internet chat rooms and suicide. *Journal of the American Academy of Child and Adolescent Psychiatry*, 43, 246–247.

BEKELMAN, J. E., HALPERN, S. D., BLANKART, C. R., BYNUM, J. P., COHEN, J., FOWLER, R., KAASA, S., KWIETNIEWSKI, L., MELBERG, H. O., ONWUTEAKA-PHILIPSEN, B., OOSTERVELD-VLUG, M., PRING, A., SCHREYÖGG, J., ULRICH, C. M., VERNE, J., WUNSCH, H. & EMANUEL, E. J. 2016. Comparison of site of death, health care utilization, and hospital expenditures for patients dying with cancer in 7 developed countries. *JAMA – Journal of the American Medical Association*, 315, 272–283.

BELLACK, A. S. 2006. Scientific and consumer models of recovery in schizophrenia: concordance, contrasts, and implications. *Schizophrenia Bulletin*, 32, 432–442.

BENATAR, D. 2020. Suicide is sometimes rational and morally defensible. In CHOLBI, M. & TIMMERMAN, T. (eds.) *Exploring the Philosophy of Death and Dying*. New York: Routledge.

BERNIER, G., MOHAMED AHMED, S. & BUSBY, C. 2020. Cost estimate for bill C-7 'medical assistance in dying'. Ottawa: Office of The Parliamentary Budget Officer.

BONGAR, B. M. 2002. *The Suicidal Patient: Clinical and Legal Standards of Care*. Washington, DC: American Psychological Association.

BOOTH, J. 2005. St Valentine's day mass suicide pact fears. *The Time*, 14 February.

BORECKY, A., THOMSEN, C. & DUBOV, A. 2019. Reweighing the ethical tradeoffs in the involuntary hospitalization of suicidal patients. *American Journal of Bioethics*, 19, 71–83.

BORRY, P., STULTIENS, L., NYS, H., CASSIMAN, J. J. & DIERICKX, K. 2006. Presymptomatic and predictive genetic testing in minors: a systematic review of guidelines and position papers. *Clinical Genetics*, 70, 374–381.

BRAITHWAITE, J. 1989. *Crime, Shame and Reintegration*. Cambridge: Cambridge University Press.

BRAITHWAITE, J. 1993. Shame and modernity. *British Journal of Criminology*, 33, 1–18.

BRITO, E. S. & VENTURA, C. A. A. 2019. Involuntary psychiatric admission: comparative study of mental health legislation in Brazil and in England/Wales. *International Journal of Law and Psychiatry*, 64, 184–197.

BROWN, J. H., HENTELEFF, P., BARAKAT, S. & ROWE, C. J. 1986. Is it normal for terminally ill patients to desire death? *American Journal of Psychiatry*, 143, 208–211.

BUCHANAN, A. 2004. Mental capacity, legal competence and consent to treatment. *Journal of the Royal Society of Medicine*, 97, 415–420.

BUITING, H. M., GEVERS, J. K. M., RIETJENS, J. A. C., ONWUTEAKA-PHILIPSEN, B. D., VAN DER MAAS, P. J., VAN DER HEIDE, A. & VAN DELDEN, J. J. M. 2008. Dutch criteria of due care for physician-assisted dying in medical practice: a physician perspective. *Journal of Medical Ethics*, 34, e12. doi: 10.1136/jme.2008.024976.

BURNS, T. 2019. Franco Basaglia: a revolutionary reformer ignored in Anglophone psychiatry. *Lancet Psychiatry*, 6, 19–21.

BURNS, T. & FOOT, J. 2020. *Basaglia's International Legacy: From Asylum to Community*. Oxford: Oxford University Press.

BURRELL, L. V., MEHLUM, L. & QIN, P. 2018. Sudden parental death from external causes and risk of suicide in the bereaved offspring: a national study. *Journal of Psychiatric Research*, 96, 49–56.

BUSHMAN, B. J. & ANDERSON, C. A. 2001. Media violence and the American public: scientific facts versus media misinformation. *American Psychologist*, 56, 477–489.

BYCHKOVA, A. M. & RADNAYEVA, E. L. 2018. Incitement to suicide with the use of internet technologies: socio-psychological, criminological and criminal law aspects. *Russian journal of criminology*, 12, 101–115.

CAIRNS, R., MADDOCK, C., BUCHANAN, A., DAVID, A. S., HAYWARD, P., RICHARDSON, G., SZMUKLER, G. & HOTOPF, M. 2005. Prevalence and predictors of mental incapacity in psychiatric in-patients. *British Journal of Psychiatry*, 187, 379–85.

CALATI, R., FILIPPONI, C., MANSI, W., CASU, D., PEVIANI, G., GENTILE, G., TAMBUZZI, S., ZOJA, R., FORNARO, M., LOPEZ-CASTROMAN, J. & MADEDDU, F. 2021. Cancer diagnosis and suicide outcomes: umbrella review and methodological considerations. *Journal of Affective Disorders*, 295, 1201–1214.

CALLAHAN, D. 1995. *Setting Limits: Medical Goals in an Aging Society*. Washington, DC: Georgetown University Press.

CAMUS, A. 1955. *The Myth of Sisyphus and Other Essays*. New York: Vintage Books.

CANADIAN INSTITUTES OF HEALTH RESEARCH & NATURAL SCIENCES AND ENGINEERING RESEARCH COUNCIL OF CANADA & SOCIAL SCIENCES AND HUMANITIES RESEARCH COUNCIL 2018. *Tri-Council Policy Statement. Ethical Conduct for Research Involving Human Subjects.* Government of Canada.

CAPLAN, A. L. 2006. Ethical issues surrounding forced, mandated, or coerced treatment. *Journal of Substance Abuse Treatment*, 31, 117–120.

CARPINIELLO, B., VITA, A. & MENCACCI, C. 2020. *Violence and Mental Disorders.* Cham: Springer.

CARROLL, R., METCALFE, C. & GUNNELL, D. 2014. Hospital presenting self-harm and risk of fatal and non-fatal repetition: systematic review and meta-analysis. *PLoS ONE*, 9, e89944.

CARTER, G., MILNER, A., MCGILL, K., PIRKIS, J., KAPUR, N. & SPITTAL, M. J. 2017. Predicting suicidal behaviours using clinical instruments: systematic review and meta-analysis of positive predictive values for risk scales. *British Journal of Psychiatry*, 210, 387–395.

CARTER V. CANADA (ATTORNEY GENERAL) 2015 SCC 5, [2015]. *1 S.C.R. 331*. Supreme Court of Canada.

CAVANAUGH, T. A. 2006. *Double-Effect Reasoning: Doing Good and Avoiding Evil.* Oxford: Oxford University Press.

CENTERS FOR DISEASE CONTROL OFFICE OF PUBLIC HEALTH GENOMICS. 2010. *ACCE Model Process for Evaluating Genetic Tests* [Online]. The Centers for Disease Control and Prevention. Available at: https://www.cdc.gov/genomics/gtesting/acce/index.htm.

CHABRIS, C. F., LEE, J. J., CESARINI, D., BENJAMIN, D. J. & LAIBSON, D. I. 2015. The fourth law of behavior genetics. *Current Directions in Psychological Science*, 24, 304–312.

CHAIMOWITZ, G. A., GLANCY, G. D. & BLACKBURN, J. 2000. The duty to warn and protect–impact on practice. *Canadian Journal of Psychiatry*, 45, 899–904.

CHAN, M. K., BHATTI, H., MEADER, N., STOCKTON, S., EVANS, J., O'CONNOR, R. C., KAPUR, N. & KENDALL, T. 2016. Predicting suicide following self-harm: systematic review of risk factors and risk scales. *British Journal of Psychiatry*, 209, 277–283.

CHANDLER, A., COVER, R. & FITZPATRICK, S. J. 2021. Critical suicide studies, between methodology and ethics: introduction. *Health (London)*, 26, 3–9.

CHENG, Q. 2011. Are internet service providers responsible for online suicide pacts? *BMJ*, 344, d2113.

CHIN, W. Y., CHAN, K. T., LAM, C. L., WAN, E. Y. & LAM, T. P. 2015. 12-month naturalistic outcomes of depressive disorders in Hong Kong's primary care. *Family Practice*, 32, 288–296.

CHO, S. E., NA, K. S., CHO, S. J., IM, J. S. & KANG, S. G. 2016. Geographical and temporal variations in the prevalence of mental disorders in suicide: systematic review and meta-analysis. *Journal of Affective Disorders*, 190, 704–713.

CHOCHINOV, H. M., HASSARD, T., MCCLEMENT, S., HACK, T., KRISTJANSON, L. J., HARLOS, M., SINCLAIR, S. & MURRAY, A. 2008. The patient dignity inventory: a novel way of measuring dignity-related distress in palliative care. *Journal of Pain and Symptom Management*, 36, 559–571.

CHOCHINOV, H. M., BARONESS FINLAY OF LLANDAFF, HENDERSON, D., HERX, L., GALLAGHER, R., KAYA, E., ADAIR, W., CARR, K., COELHO, R., ETHANS, K., FRAZEE, C., GRANT, I., HEWITT, M., JAMA, S., JANZ, H., JOFFE, K., LINTON, M., NICHOLS, G., NICHOLS, T., PETERS, G., SHANNON, D. W., STAINTON, T., COHEN, E., HENICK, M., KELLEHER, E., KRAUSERT, S. D., MAHER, J., MISHARA, B. L., VRAKAS, G., BELANGER, N., EHMANN, T., HENRY, M., MEHDI, A., MCCORMICK, R., MONTES, M. A., SHEEHY, E., BACH, M., BEAUDRY, J.-B., CHUNG, A. M., FERRIER, C., GALLAGHER, R., LEMMENS, T. & PAGEAU, F. 2023. *Expert Witnesses Speak Out Against Bias in Medical Assistance in Dying Report*. https://static1.squarespace .com/static/61db373a8e4e00423c117825/t/640739a3f6062c0b00236 bbe/1678195107898/MAID+Report+Response+March+7+2023.pdf.

CHOO, P. Y., TAN-HO, G., DUTTA, O., PATINADAN, P. V. & HO, A. H. Y. 2020. Reciprocal dynamics of dignity in end-of-life care: a multiperspective systematic review of qualitative and mixed methods research. *American Journal of Hospice and Palliative Medicine*, 37, 385–398.

CHORON, J. 1964. *Modern Man and Mortality*. Oxford: Macmillan.

CHORON, J. 1972. *Suicide*. New York: Charles Scribner's Sons.

CHOY, C. H. 2017. Suicide in palliative care setting. *Annals of Palliative Medicine*, 6, S264–S265.

CLARKE, D. M. 1999. Autonomy, rationality and the wish to die. *Journal of Medical Ethics*, 25, 457–462.

CLEARY, A. 2019. The meaning and context of suicidal action. In CLEARY, A. (ed.) *The Gendered Landscape of Suicide: Masculinities, Emotions, and Culture*. Cham: Springer.

COHEN-ALMAGOR, R. 2009. Euthanasia policy and practice in Belgium: critical observations and suggestions for improvement. *Issues in Law and Medicine*, 24, 187–218.

COHEN-ALMAGOR, R. 2015. First do no harm: intentionally shortening lives of patients without their explicit request in Belgium. *Journal of Medical Ethics*, 41, 625–629.

COLEMAN, A. M. E. 2021. Police emergency commitment powers in cases of persons experiencing mental health crisis in 'public spaces': review of the commitment process in England and Wales, in comparison to the practice in the United States of America (USA). *Open Journal of Psychiatry*, 11, 219–228.

COMMISSION FÉDÉRALE DE CONTRÔLE ET D'ÉVALUATION DE L'EUTHANASIE 2020. Neuvième rapport aux Chambres législatives 2018-2019. Brussels: Santé publique, Sécurité de la Chaîne alimentaire et Environnement.

COMMISSION SPÉCIALE SUR LA QUESTION DE MOURIR DANS LA DIGNITÉ 2012. Consultation générale et auditions publiques sur la question de mourir dans la dignité. Montreal: Assemblé Nationale du Québec.

COMMONWEALTH OF AUSTRALIA 2005. Criminal Code Amendment (Suicide Related Material Offences) Act. Australia Criminal Code Act 1995 2005.

COOLEY, D. R. 2013. A Kantian care ethics suicide duty. *International Journal of Law and Psychiatry*, 36, 366–373.

COOLEY, D. R. 2015a. A duty to suicide. In COOLEY, D. R. (ed.) *Death's Values and Obligations: A Pragmatic Framework*. Dordrecht: Springer.

COOLEY, D. R. 2015b. Justifying a duty to suicide. *Ethics, Medicine and Public Health*, 1, 532–542.

CORNEL, M. C., VAN EL, C. G. & BORRY, P. 2014. The challenge of implementing genetic tests with clinical utility while avoiding unsound applications. *Journal of Community Genetics*, 5, 7–12.

COUNCIL FOR INTERNATIONAL ORGANIZATIONS OF MEDICAL SCIENCES (CIOMS) 2016. *International Ethical Guidelines for Biomedical Research Involving Human Subjects*. Prepared by the Council for International Organizations of Medical Sciences (CIOMS) in collaboration with the World Health Organization (WHO).

CREPEAU-HOBSON, M. F. & LEECH, N. L. 2014. The impact of exposure to peer suicidal self-directed violence on youth suicidal behavior: a critical review of the literature. *Suicide and Life-Threatening Behavior*, 44, 58–77.

CROWE, M. & CARLYLE, D. 2003. Deconstructing risk assessment and management in mental health nursing. *Journal of Advanced Nursing*, 43, 19–27.

D66. 2016. *Pia Dijkstra publiceert wetsinitiatief waardig levenseinde [Pia Dijkstra publishes law initiative dignifiedend of life]* [Online]. Available at: https://d66 .nl/wet-voltooid-leven-pia-dijkstra/.

DAVIS, D. S. 2015. VII. Feminism and suicide in the face of dementia. *Feminism and Psychology*, 25, 131–136.

DAWSON, J. & SZMUKLER, G. 2006. Fusion of mental health and incapacity legislation. *British Journal of Psychiatry*, 188, 504–509.

DAWSON, J. P. 1960. Negotiorum gestio: the altruistic intermeddler. *Harvard Law Review*, 74, 817.

DE BOER, M. E., DEPLA, M., DEN BREEJEN, M., SLOTTJE, P., ONWUTEAKA-PHILIPSEN, B. D. & HERTOGH, C. 2019. Pressure in dealing with requests for euthanasia or assisted suicide: experiences of general practitioners. *Journal of Medical Ethics*, 45, 425–429.

/DEES, M., VERNOOIJ-DASSEN, M., DEKKERS, W. & VAN WEEL, C. 2010. Unbearable suffering of patients with a request for euthanasia or physician-assisted suicide: an integrative review. *Psycho-Oncology*, 19, 339–352.

DEGENHOLTZ, H. B., PARKER, L. S. & REYNOLDS, C. F. 2002. Trial design and informed consent for a clinic-based study with a treatment as usual control arm. *Ethics and Behavior*, 12, 43–62.

DEJONG, T. M., OVERHOLSER, J. C. & STOCKMEIER, C. A. 2010. Apples to oranges? A direct comparison between suicide attempters and suicide completers. *Journal of Affective Disorders*, 124, 90–97.

DEVANDAS-AGUILAR, C. & UNITED NATION HUMAN RIGHTS COUNCIL SPECIAL RAPPORTEUR ON THE RIGHTS OF PERSONS WITH DISABILITIES 2019. *Visit to Canada: Report of the Special Rapporteur on the Rights of Persons with Disabilities. United Nation Human Rights Council Special Rapporteur on the Rights of Persons with Disabilities.*

DISHNEAU, D. 2015. Lazzaric Caldwell suicide attempt conviction reversed. *Huffington Post*, 7 June.

DJELANTIK, A., SMID, G. E., MROZ, A., KLEBER, R. J. & BOELEN, P. A. 2020. The prevalence of prolonged grief disorder in bereaved individuals following unnatural losses: systematic review and meta regression analysis. *Journal of Affective Disorders*, 265, 146–156.

DOBSON, R. 1999. Internet sites may encourage suicide. *British Medical Journal*, 319, 337.

DONNELLY, M. 2010. *Healthcare Decision-Making and the Law: Autonomy, Capacity and the Limits of Liberalism*. Cambridge: Cambridge University Press.

DRAPER, B., MACCUSPIE-MOORE, C. & BRODATY, H. 1998. Suicidal ideation and the 'wish to die' in dementia patients: the role of depression. *Age Ageing*, 27, 503–507.

DRAPER, J., MURPHY, G., VEGA, E., COVINGTON, D. W. & MCKEON, R. 2015. Helping callers to the National Suicide Prevention Lifeline who are at imminent risk of suicide: the importance of active engagement, active rescue, and collaboration between crisis and emergency services. *Suicide and Life-Threatening Behavior*, 45, 261–270.

DRION, H. 1992. *Het zelfgewilde einde van oude mensen*. Amsterdam: Balans.

DUBLIN, L. I. & BUNZEL, B. 1933. *To Be or Not to Be: A Study of Suicide*. New York: Harrison Smith and Robert Haas.

DUPRE, C. 2009. Unlocking human dignity: towards a theory for the 21st century. *European Human Rights Law Review*, 2, 190–205.

DURKHEIM, E. 1985. *Le suicide*. Paris: Presses universitaires de France.

DURLAK, J. A. 1979. Comparative effectiveness of paraprofessional and professional helpers. *Psychological Bulletin*, 86, 80–92.

DWORKIN, G. 1988. *The Theory and Practice of Autonomy*. New York: Cambridge University Press.

DWORKIN, R. 1986. Autonomy and the demented self. *The Milbank Quarterly*, 64, 4–16.

DYCK, E. 2011. Dismantling the asylum and charting new pathways into the community: mental health care in twentieth century Canada. *Social history*, 44, 181–196.

ECONOMIST INTELLIGENCE UNIT 2010. *The Quality of Death: Ranking End-of-life Care Across the World*. https://www.dgpalliativmedizin.de/images/stories/the_quality_of_death1a.pdf.

EISENBERG, M. A. 2002. The duty to rescue in contract law. *Fordham Law Review*, 71. Available at: https://ir.lawnet.fordham.edu/flr/vol71/iss3/3.

EMANUEL, E. J., ONWUTEAKA-PHILIPSEN, B. D., URWIN, J. W. & COHEN, J. 2016. Attitudes and practices of euthanasia and physician-assisted suicide in the United States, Canada, and Europe. *Journal of the American Medical Association*, 316, 79–90.

ENGLAND 1961. Suicide Act 1961. *12*. Available at: https://www.legislation.gov.uk/ukpga/Eliz2/9-10/60.

EPICTETUS 1910. *The Moral Discourses of Epictetus*. London: J. M. Dent & Sons.

ETINSON, A. 2020. What's so special about human dignity? *Philosophy & Public Affairs*, 48, 353–381.

EUROPEAN UNION 1999. *Multiannual Community Action Plan on Promoting Safer Use of the Internet by Combating Illegal and Harmful Content on Global Networks*. Brussels: European Union.

EVANS, R., WHITE, J., TURLEY, R., SLATER, T., MORGAN, H., STRANGE, H. & SCOURFIELD, J. 2017. Comparison of suicidal ideation, suicide attempt and suicide in children and young people in care and non-care populations: systematic review and meta-analysis of prevalence. *Children and Youth Services Review*, 82, 122–129.

EVENBLIJ, K., PASMAN, H. R. W., PRONK, R. & ONWUTEAKA-PHILIPSEN, B. D. 2019. Euthanasia and physician-assisted suicide in patients suffering from psychiatric disorders: a cross-sectional study exploring the experiences of Dutch psychiatrists. *BMC Psychiatry*, 19, 74.

FAGOT-LARGEAULT, A., LÉNA, P. & COMBES, F. O. 2021. *Ontologie du devenir: l'évolution, l'univers et le temps*. Paris: Odile Jacob.

FAVARO, A., ST. PHILIP, E. & SLAUGHTER, G. 2019. *Family says B.C. man with history of depression wasn't fit for assisted death* [Online]. CTV News. Available at: https://www.ctvnews.ca/health/family-says-b-c-man-with-history-of-depression-wasn-t-fit-for-assisted-death-1.4609016.

FEINBERG, J. 1980. *Rights, Justice, and the Bounds of Liberty: Essays in Social Philosophy*. Princeton: Princeton University Press.

FELDBRUGGE, F. J. M. 1965. Good and bad samaritans: a comparative survey of criminal law provisions concerning failure to rescue. *American Journal of Comparative Law*, 14, 630–657.

FERRAND, E., DREYFUS, J. F., CHASTRUSSE, M., ELLIEN, F., LEMAIRE, F. & FISCHLER, M. 2012. Evolution of requests to hasten death among patients managed by palliative care teams in France: a multicentre cross-sectional survey (DemandE). *European Journal of Cancer*, 48, 368–376.

FINLAY, I. G. & GEORGE, R. 2011. Legal physician-assisted suicide in Oregon and the Netherlands: evidence concerning the impact on patients in vulnerable groups – another perspective on Oregon's data. *Journal of Medical Ethics*, 37, 171–174.

FISHER, C. B., PEARSON, J. L., KIM, S. & REYNOLDS, C. F. 2002. Ethical issues in including suicidal individuals in clinical research. *IRB Ethics & Human Research*, 24, 9–14.

FISTEIN, E. C., HOLLAND, A. J., CLARE, I. C. & GUNN, M. J. 2009. A comparison of mental health legislation from diverse Commonwealth jurisdictions. *International Journal of Law and Psychiatry*, 32, 147–155.

FITZPATRICK, S. J. 2021. The moral and political economy of suicide prevention. *Journal of Sociology*, 58, 113–129.

FOOT, J. 2015. *The Man who Closed the Asylums: Franco Basaglia and the Revolution in Mental Health Care*. London: Verso.

FORCIGNANÒ, V. 2021. *Disability Is Not a Reason to Sanction Medically Assisted Dying – UN Experts*. Geneva: The Office of the High Commissioner for Human Rights.

FOSTER, C. 2019. Dignity in medical law. In PHILLIPS, A. M., CAMPOS, T. C. D. & HERRING, J. (eds.) *Philosophical Foundations of Medical Law*. Oxford: Oxford University Press.

FOTION, N., KASHNIKOV, B. & LEKEA, J. K. 2007. *Epz Terrorism: The New World Disorder*. London: Bloomsbury.

FOUCAULT, M. 1976. *Histoire de la sexualite*. Paris: Gallimard.

FREEDMAN, B. 1987. Equipoise and the ethics of clinical research. *New England Journal of Medicine*, 317, 141–145.

FREI, A., SCHENKER, T. A., FINZEN, A., KRÄUCHI, K., DITTMANN, V. & HOFFMANN-RICHTER, U. 2001. Assisted suicide as conducted by a 'right-to-die'-society in Switzerland: a descriptive analysis of 43 consecutive cases. *Swiss Medical Weekly*, 131, 375–380.

FRIEDLANDER, G. 1915. *Laws and Customs of Israel*. London: Vallentine and Sons.

FU, Q., HEATH, A. C., BUCHOLZ, K. K., NELSON, E. C., GLOWINSKI, A. L., GOLDBERG, J., LYONS, M. J., TSUANG, M. T., JACOB, T., TRUE, M. R. & EISEN, S. A. 2002. A twin study of genetic and environmental influences on suicidality in men. *Psychological Medicine*, 32, 11–24.

GEIST, M. A. 2002. *Internet Law in Canada*, 3rd Edition. Concord: Captus Press.

GIJSWIJT-HOFSTRA, M. 2005. *Psychiatric Cultures Compared: Psychiatry and Mental Health Care in the Twentieth Century: Comparisons and Approaches*. Amsterdam: Amsterdam University Press.

GOMES, B., CALANZANI, N., CURIALE, V., MCCRONE, P. & HIGGINSON, I. J. 2013. Effectiveness and cost-effectiveness of home palliative care services for adults with advanced illness and their caregivers. *Cochrane Database of Systematic Reviews*, CD007760.

GOODWIN, S. 1997. *Comparative Mental Health Policy: From Institutional to Community Care*. London: Sage.

GOVERNMENT OF THE UNITED KINGDOM 1957. *Homicide Act*. London: Government of the United Kingdom.

GRAY, J. E., MCSHERRY, B. M., O'REILLY, R. L. & WELLER, P. J. 2010. Australian and Canadian Mental Health Acts compared. *Australian and New Zealand Journal of Psychiatry*, 44, 1126–1131.

GRISSO, T., APPELBAUM, P. S. & HILL-FOTOUHI, C. 1997. The MacCAT-T: a clinical tool to assess patients' capacities to make treatment decisions. *Psychiatric Services*, 48, 1415–1419.

GROTH, T. & BOCCIO, D. E. 2019. psychologists' willingness to provide services to individuals at risk of suicide. *Suicide and Life-Threatening Behavior*, 49, 1241–1254.

HAERPFER, C., INGLEHART, R., MORENO, A., WELZEL, C., KIZILOVA, K., DIEZ-MEDRANO, J., LAGOS, M., NORRIS, P., PONARIN, E. & PURANEN, B. 2022. *World Values Survey: Round Seven – Country-Pooled Datafile Version 5.0*. Madrid, & Vienna: JD Systems Institute & WVSA Secretariat. doi: 10.14281/18241.20.

HAGENKORD, J., FUNKE, B., QIAN, E., HEGDE, M., JACOBS, K. B., FERBER, M., LEBO, M., BUCHANAN, A. & BICK, D. 2020. Design and reporting considerations for genetic screening tests. *Journal of Molecular Diagnostics*, 22, 599–609.

HALE, B., GORMAN, P., BARRETT, R. & JONES, J. 2017. *Mental Health Law*. London: Sweet & Maxwell.

HALLECK, S. L. 2012. *Law in the Practice of Psychiatry: A Handbook for Clinicians*. Cham: Springer.

HARDING, A. 2004. BBC News. *Japan's Internet 'suicide clubs'*.

HARDWIG, J. 1997a. Dying at the right time: reflections on (un)assisted suicide. In LAFOLLETTE, H. (ed.) *Ethics in Practice: An Anthology*. Oxford: Blackwell.

HARDWIG, J. 1997b. Is there a duty to die? *The Hastings Center Report*, 27, 34–42.

HARDY, J. & SINGLETON, A. 2009. Genomewide association studies and human disease. *New England Journal of Medicine*, 360, 1759–1768.

HARTOG, I. D., ZOMERS, M. L., VAN THIEL, G., LEGET, C., SACHS, A. P. E., UITERWAAL, C., VAN DEN BERG, V. & VAN WIJNGAARDEN, E. 2020. Prevalence and characteristics of older adults with a persistent death wish without severe illness: a large cross-sectional survey. *BMC Geriatrics*, 20, 342.

HASSAN, N. 2001. Letter from Gaza: an arsenal of believers. *The New Yorker*.

HATTIE, J. A. & HANSFORD, B. C. 1984. Meta-analysis: a reflection on problems. *Australian Journal of Psychology*, 36, 239–254.

HAUSWIRTH, A. G., GEORGE, H. C. & LOMEN-HOERTH, C. 2021. ALS patient and caregiver attitudes toward physician-hastened death in California. *Muscle Nerve*, 64, 428–434.

HAWKING, S. W. 2015. *Stephen Hawking: 'Technology seems to drive inequality.'* [Online]. World Economic Forum. Available at: https://www.weforum.org/agenda/2015/10/stephen-hawking-technology-seems-to-drive-ever-increasing-inequality/.

HAWRYLUCK, L. 2017. Issues of vulnerability and equality: the emerging need for court evaluations of physicians' fiduciary duties in high stakes end-of-life decisions. *Health Law Canada*, 37, 86–95.

HAWTON, K., ARENSMAN, E., TOWNSEND, E., BREMNER, S., FELDMAN, E., GOLDNEY, R., GUNNELL, D., HAZELL, P., VAN HEERINGEN, K., HOUSE, A., OWENS, D., SAKINOFSKY, I. & TRÄSKMAN-BENDZ, L. 1998. Deliberate self harm: systematic review of efficacy of psychosocial and pharmacological treatments in preventing repetition. *British Medical Journal*, 317, 441–447.

HAWTON, K. & WILLIAMS, K. 2001. The connection between media and suicidal behavior warrants serious attention. *Crisis*, 22, 137–140.

HAYDEN, A. 2000. Imposing criminal and civil penalties for failing to help another: are Good Samaritan laws good ideas. *New England International and Comparative Law Annual*, 6, 27.

HELD, V. 1996. *Feminist Morality Transforming Culture, Society, and Politics.* Chicago: The University of Chicago Press.

HENDIN, H., LITMAN, R., MOTTO, J., PARDES, H. & PFEFFER, C. 1985. Report of the National Conference on Youth Suicide. US Dept of Health and Human Services. https://www.ojp.gov/pdffiles1/Digitization/108311NCJRS.pdf.

HENDRY, M., PASTERFIELD, D., LEWIS, R., CARTER, B., HODGSON, D. & WILKINSON, C. 2013. Why do we want the right to die? A systematic review of the international literature on the views of patients, carers and the public on assisted dying. *Palliative Medicine*, 27, 13–26.

HENGARTNER, M. P., AMENDOLA, S., KAMINSKI, J. A., KINDLER, S., BSCHOR, T. & PLÖDERL, M. 2021. Suicide risk with selective serotonin reuptake inhibitors and other new-generation antidepressants in adults: a systematic review and meta-analysis of observational studies. *Journal of Epidemiology and Community Health*. doi: 10.1136/jech-2020-214611.

HENSEL, J. 2020. How a new standard of care can make social media companies better 'Good Samaritans.' *Minnesota Law Review*, 105, 1453–1483.

HERRING, J. 2022. *The Right to Be Protected from Committing Suicide.* Oxford: Hart Publishing.

HETRICK, S. E., MCKENZIE, J. E., BAILEY, A. P., SHARMA, V., MOLLER, C. I., BADCOCK, P. B., COX, G. R., MERRY, S. N. & MEADER, N. 2021. New generation antidepressants for depression in children and adolescents: a network meta-analysis. *Cochrane Database of Systematic Reviews*, 5, CD013674.

HIGGINS, D. M., MARTIN, A. M., BAKER, D. G., VASTERLING, J. J. & RISBROUGH, V. 2018. The relationship between chronic pain and neurocognitive function: a systematic review. *Clinical Journal of Pain*, 34, 262–275.

HIRSCHHORN, J. N. & DALY, M. J. 2005. Genome-wide association studies for common diseases and complex traits. *Nature Reviews Genetics*, 6, 95–108.

HO, A. O. 2014. Suicide: rationality and responsibility for life. *Canadian Journal of Psychiatry/Revue canadienne de psychiatrie*, 59, 141–147.

HOLMSTRAND, C., RAHM HALLBERG, I., SAKS, K., LEINO-KILPI, H., RENOM GUITERAS, A., VERBEEK, H., ZABALEGUI, A., SUTCLIFFE, C. & LETHIN, C. 2021. Associated factors of suicidal ideation among older persons with dementia living at home in eight European countries. *Aging and Mental Health*, 25, 1730–1739.

HOLZMAN, T. J. 2021. The final act: an ethical analysis of Pia Dijkstra's *Euthanasia for a Completed Life*. *Journal of Bioethical Inquiry*, 18, 165–175.

HUA, P., BUGEJA, L. & MAPLE, M. 2019. A systematic review on the relationship between childhood exposure to external cause parental death, including suicide, on subsequent suicidal behaviour. *Journal of Affective Disorders*, 257, 723–734.

HUME, D. 1894. *An Essay on Suicide*. London, R. Forder.

HUMPHRY, D. 1986. The case for rational suicide. *Euthanasia Review*, 1, 172–176.

HUMPHRY, D. 1991. *Final Exit: The Practicalities of Self-deliverance and Assisted Suicide for the Dying*. Eugene: Hemlock Society.

IKUNAGA, A., NATH, S. R. & SKINNER, K. A. 2013. Internet suicide in Japan: a qualitative content analysis of a suicide bulletin board. *Transcultural Psychiatry*, 50, 280–302.

INNES, J. 2003. Coroner calls for police watch on web chat rooms. *The Scotsman*, 1 October.

ISTITUZIONE DEL SERVIZIO SANITARIO NAZIONALE 1978. *Accertamenti e trattamenti sanitari volontari e obbligatori*.

JIANG, F. F., XU, H. L., LIAO, H. Y. & ZHANG, T. 2017. Analysis of internet suicide pacts reported by the media in mainland China. *Crisis*, 38, 36–43.

JOBES, D. A. & BERMAN, A. L. 1993. Suicide and malpractice liability: assessing and revising policies, procedures, and practice in outpatient settings. *Professional Psychology: Research and Practice*, 24, 91–99.

JONES-BONOFIGLIO, K. 2020. *Health Care Ethics Through the Lens of Moral Distress*. Cham: Springer.

JOO, S. H., WANG, S. M., KIM, T. W., SEO, H. J., JEONG, J. H., HAN, J. H. & HONG, S. C. 2016. Factors associated with suicide completion: a comparison between suicide attempters and completers. *Asia-Pacific Psychiatry*, 8, 80–86.

JUDGEMENTS OF THE SUPREME COURT OF CANADA 1993. *Rodriguez v. British Columbia (Attorney General)*.

KAHAN, D. M. 1996. What do alternative sanctions mean? *The University of Chicago Law Review*, 63, 591–653.

KAHAN, D. M. 2002. Shaming punishments. In DRESSLER, J. (ed.) *Encyclopedia of Crime & Justice*. New York: Macmillan Reference USA.

KALLMANN, F. J. 1953. *Heredity in Health and Mental Disorder: Principles of Psychiatric Genetics in the Light of Comparative Twin Studies*. Oxford: W. W. Norton.

KAMISAR, Y. 1998. The future of physician-assisted suicide. *Trial*, 34, 48–53.

KANT, I. 1949. *Fundamental Principles of the Metaphysic of Morals*. New York: Liberal Arts Press (Original work published 1785).

KANT, I. 1963. *Lectures on Ethics*. Indianapolis: Hackett Publishing Company.

KASTENBAUM, R. 2000. *The Psychology of Death*. New York: Springer.

KESSLER, R. C., BOSSARTE, R. M., LUEDTKE, A., ZASLAVSKY, A. M. & ZUBIZARRETA, J. R. 2020. Suicide prediction models: a critical review of recent research with recommendations for the way forward. *Molecular Psychiatry*, 25, 168–179.

KHATTAB, M. 2016. 4:29, 4:30. An-Nisa. In KHATTAB M. (Transl. and ed.) *The Clear Quran*. Book of Signs Foundation.

KHAZEM, L. R. 2018. Physical disability and suicide: recent advancements in understanding and future directions for consideration. *Current Opinion in Psychology*, 22, 18–22.

KISELY, S. R. & CAMPBELL, L. A. 2015. Compulsory community and involuntary outpatient treatment for people with severe mental disorders. *Schizophrenia Bulletin*, 41, 542–543.

KLINGEMANN, H., SOBELL, M. B. & SOBELL, L. C. 2010. Continuities and changes in self-change research. *Addiction*, 105, 1510–1518.

KNIPE, D., WILLIAMS, A. J., HANNAM-SWAIN, S., UPTON, S., BROWN, K., BANDARA, P., CHANG, S. S. & KAPUR, N. 2019. Psychiatric morbidity and suicidal behaviour in low- and middle-income countries: a systematic review and meta-analysis. *PLoS Medicine*, 16, e1002905.

KNOLL IV, J. L. 2019. Suicide prohibition: shame, blame, or social aim? In HALDIPUR, C. V., KNOLL IV, J. L. & VD LUFT, E. (eds.) *Thomas Szasz: An Appraisal of his Legacy*. New York: Oxford University Press.

LAWRENCE, R. E. & APPELBAUM, P. S. 2011. Genetic testing in psychiatry: a review of attitudes and beliefs. *Psychiatry: Interpersonal and Biological Processes*, 74, 315–331.

LECKY, W. E. H. 1869. *History of European Morals from Augustus to Charlemagne, Vol. 2*. New York: D. Appleton & Company.

LEE, S. Y. & KWON, Y. 2018. Twitter as a place where people meet to make suicide pacts. *Public Health*, 159, 21–26.

LERNER, B. H. & CAPLAN, A. L. 2015. Euthanasia in Belgium and the Netherlands: on a slippery slope? *JAMA Internal Medicine*, 175, 1640–1641.

LESTER, D. 1992. Decriminalization of suicide in Canada and suicide rates. *Psychological Reports*, 71, 738.

LEVENE, I. & PARKER, M. 2011. Prevalence of depression in granted and refused requests for euthanasia and assisted suicide: a systematic review. *Journal of Medical Ethics*, 37, 205–211.

LEWIS, N. A. 2005. Guantánamo prisoners go on hunger strike. *The New York Times*, 18 September.

LILLEHAMMER, H. 2002. Voluntary euthanasia and the logical slippery slope argument. *The Cambridge Law Journal*, 61, 545–550.

LIN, H. C., WU, C. H. & LEE, H. C. 2009. Risk factors for suicide following hospital discharge among cancer patients. *Psychooncology*, 18, 1038–1044.

LINDEN, A. M. 1972. Rescuers and Good Samaritans. *Alberta Law Review*, 10, 72–88.

LINTHICUM, K. P., SCHAFER, K. M. & RIBEIRO, J. D. 2019. Machine learning in suicide science: applications and ethics. *Behavioral Sciences & the Law*, 37, 214–222.

LIU, R. T., BETTIS, A. H. & BURKE, T. A. 2020. Characterizing the phenomenology of passive suicidal ideation: a systematic review and meta-analysis of its prevalence, psychiatric comorbidity, correlates, and comparisons with active suicidal ideation. *Psychological Medicine*, 50, 367–383.

LUTZ, P. E., MECHAWAR, N. & TURECKI, G. 2017. Neuropathology of suicide: recent findings and future directions. *Molecular Psychiatry*, 22, 1395–1412.

LYSSENKO, V. & LAAKSO, M. 2013. Genetic screening for the risk of type 2 diabetes: worthless or valuable? *Diabetes Care*, 36, S120–S126.

MACINTYRE, V. G., MANSELL, W., PRATT, D. & TAI, S. J. 2021. The psychological pathway to suicide attempts: a strategy of control without awareness. *Frontiers in Psychology*, 12, 588683.

MACKENZIE, C. & STOLJAR, N. 2000. *Relational Autonomy: Feminist Perspectives on Autonomy, Agency, and the Social Self*. Oxford: Oxford University Press.

MACKLIN, R. 1999. *Against Relativism: Cultural Diversity and the Search for Ethical Universals in Medicine*. New York: Oxford University Press.

MACSHERRY, B. 2010. *Rethinking Rights-based Mental Health Laws*. Oxford: Hart.

MAESSEN, M., VELDINK, J. H., VAN DEN BERG, L. H., SCHOUTEN, H. J., VAN DER WAL, G. & ONWUTEAKA-PHILIPSEN, B. D. 2010. Requests for euthanasia: origin of suffering in ALS, heart failure, and cancer patients. *Journal of Neurology*, 257, 1192–1198.

MAIDA, A. 2017. *Online and on All Fronts. Russia's Assault on Freedom of Expression*. [Online]. Human Rights Watch. Available at: https://www.hrw.org/report/2017/07/18/online-and-all-fronts/russias-assault-freedom-expression.

MANN, J. J., CURRIER, D., STANLEY, B., OQUENDO, M. A., AMSEL, L. V. & ELLIS, S. P. 2006. Can biological tests assist prediction of suicide in mood disorders? *International Journal of Neuropsychopharmacology*, 9, 465–474.

MARCOUX, I., BOIVIN, A., ARSENAULT, C., TOUPIN, M. & YOUSSEF, J. 2015. Health care professionals' comprehension of the legal status of end-of-life practices in Quebec: study of clinical scenarios. *Canadian Family Physician*, 61, e196–e203.

MARCOUX, I., MISHARA, B. L. & DURAND, C. 2007. Confusion between euthanasia and other end-of-life decisions: influences on public opinion poll results. *Canadian Journal of Public Health*, 98, 235–239.

MARIS, R. 1982. Rational suicide: an impoverished self-transformation. *Suicide and Life-Threatening Behavior*, 12, 4–16.

MARIS, R. W. 1992. Summary and conclusions: What have we learned about suicide assessment and prediction? In MARIS, R. W., BERMAN, A. L., MALTSBERGER, J. T., YUFIR, R. I. (eds.) *Assessment and Prediction of Suicide*. New York: Guilford Press.

MASSARO, T. M. 1991. Shame, culture, and American criminal law. *Michigan Law Review*, 89, 1880–1944.

MAYO, D. J. 1983. Contemporary philosophical literature on suicide: a review. *Suicide and Life-Threatening Behavior*, 13, 313–345.

MAYO, D. J. 1986. The concept of rational suicide. *Journal of Medicine and Philosophy*, 11, 143–155.

MCGOWAN, P. O., SASAKI, A., D'ALESSIO, A. C., DYMOV, S., LABONTÉ, B., SZYF, M., TURECKI, G. & MEANEY, M. J. 2009. Epigenetic regulation of the glucocorticoid receptor in human brain associates with childhood abuse. *Nature Neuroscience*, 12, 342–348.

MCHUGH, C. M., CORDEROY, A., RYAN, C. J., HICKIE, I. B. & LARGE, M. M. 2019. Association between suicidal ideation and suicide: meta-analyses of odds ratios, sensitivity, specificity and positive predictive value. *BJPsych Open*, 5, e18. doi: 10.1192/bjo.2018.88.

MCPHERSON, E. 2006. Genetic diagnosis and testing in clinical practice. *Clinical Medicine & Research*, 4, 123–129.

MCSHERRY, B. 2012. Legal capacity under the Convention on the Rights of Persons with Disabilities. *Journal of Law and Medicine*, 20, 22–27.

MEHARG, D. P., NAANYU, V., RAMBALDINI, B., CLARKE, M. J., LACEY, C., JEBASINGH, F., LOPEZ-JARAMILLO, P., GOULD, G. S., ACEVES, B., ALISON, J. A., CHAITON, M., CHEN, J., GONZALEZ-SALAZAR, F., GOODYEAR-SMITH, F., GWYNNE, K. G., LEE, K. S., MACKAY, D., MAPLE-BROWN, L., MISHARA, B. L., NIGENDA, G., RAMANI-CHANDER, A., SHERWOOD, S. G., THOMAS, N., THRIFT, A. G. & ANDERSON, M. 2023. The Global Alliance for Chronic Diseases researchers' statement on non-communicable disease research with Indigenous peoples. *Lancet Global Health*, 11, e324–e326.

MEHLUM, L. 2000. The internet, suicide, and suicide prevention. *Crisis*, 21, 186–188.

MICCINESI, G., CROCETTI, E., BENVENUTI, A. & PACI, E. 2004. Suicide mortality is decreasing among cancer patients in Central Italy. *European Journal of Cancer*, 40, 1053–1057.

MILLER, D., EARLEY, P. & HANSON, A. 2018. *Committed: The Battle over Involuntary Psychiatric Care*. Baltimore: John Hopkins University Press.

MILLER, D. N. 2019. Suicidal behavior in children: issues and implications for elementary schools. *Contemporary School Psychology*, 23, 357–366.

MINKOWITZ, T. 2006. The United Nations Convention on the Rights of Persons with Disabilities and the Right to Be Free from Nonconsensual Psychiatric Interventions Symposium: The United Nations Convention on the Rights of Persons with Disabilities. *Syracuse Journal of International Law and Commerce*, 2, 405–428.

MISHARA, B. L. 1998. 27. The right to die and the right to live: perspectives on euthanasia and assisted suicide. In LEENAARS, A., SAKINOFSKY, I., WENCKSTERN, S., DYCK, R., KRAL, M. & BLAND, R. (eds.) *Suicide in Canada*. Toronto: University of Toronto Press.

MISHARA, B. 1999a. Conceptions of death and suicide in children ages 6–12 and their implications for suicide prevention. *Suicide and Life Threatening Behavior*, 29, 105–118.

MISHARA, B. L. 1999b. Synthesis of research and evidence on factors affecting the desire of terminally ill or seriously chronically ill persons to hasten death. *Omega: Journal of Death and Dying*, 39, 1–70.

MISHARA, B. L. 2002. Suicide types: rational suicide. In KASTENBAUM, R. & LEAMAN, O. (eds.) *Macmillan Encyclopedia of Death and Dying*. Farmington Hills: Gale, Cengage Learning.

MISHARA, B. 2003. Des pratiques novatrices pour la prévention du suicide au Québec: un défi de société. *Santé mentale au Québec*, XXVIII, 111–125.

MISHARA, B. L. 2013. force-feeding is only part of an ethical intervention. room for debate. *The New York Times*.

MISHARA, B. L. & DARGIS, L. 2019. Systematic comparison of recommendations for safe messaging about suicide in public communications. *Journal of Affective Disorders*, 244, 124–154.

MISHARA, B. L. & KERKHOF, A. J. F. M. 2018. Canadian and Dutch doctors' roles in assistance in dying. *Canadian Journal of Public Health*, 109, 726–728.

MISHARA, B. & TOUSIGNANT, M. 2004. *Comprendre le suicide*. Montréal: Presses de l'Université de Montréal.

MISHARA, B. L. & WEISSTUB, D. N. 2005. Ethical and legal issues in suicide research. *International Journal of Law and Psychiatry*, 28, 23–41.

MISHARA, B. L. & WEISSTUB, D. N. 2007. Ethical, legal, and practical issues in the control and regulation of suicide promotion and assistance over the internet. *Suicide and Life-Threatening Behavior*, 37, 58–65.

MISHARA, B. L. & WEISSTUB, D. N. 2010. Resolving ethical dilemmas in suicide prevention: the case of telephone helpline rescue policies. *Suicide and Life-Threatening Behavior*, 40, 159–169.

MISHARA, B. L. & WEISSTUB, D. N. 2013. Premises and evidence in the rhetoric of assisted suicide and euthanasia. *International Journal of Law and Psychiatry*, 36, 427–435.

MISHARA, B. L. & WEISSTUB, D. N. 2015. Legalization of euthanasia in Quebec, Canada as 'medical aid in dying': a case study in social marketing, changing mores and legal maneuvering. *Ethics, Medicine and Public Health*, 1, 450–455.

MISHARA, B. L. & WEISSTUB, D. N. 2016. The legal status of suicide: a global review. *International Journal of Law and Psychiatry*, 44, 54–74.

MISHARA, B. L. & WEISSTUB, D. N. 2018. Is suicide prevention an absolute? *Crisis*, 39, 313–317.

MISHARA, B. L. & WEISSTUB, D. N. 2021. Genetic testing for suicide risk assessment: theoretical premises, research challenges and ethical concerns. *Preventive Medicine*, 152, 106685.

MISHARA, B. L. & WEISSTUB, D. N. 2022. From involuntary incarceration to medically assisted suicide: mental illness, suicide and autonomous judgement. *Ethics, Medicine and Public Health*, 23, 100779.

MISHARA, B. L., CHAGNON, F., DAIGLE, M., BALAN, B., RAYMOND, S., MARCOUX, I., BARDON, C., CAMPBELL, J. K. & BERMAN, A. 2007. Comparing models of helper behavior to actual practice in telephone crisis intervention: a silent monitoring study of calls to the U.S. 1-800-SUICIDE network. *Suicide and Life-Threatening Behavior*, 37, 291–307.

MISHARA, B. L., DAIGLE, M., BARDON, C., CHAGNON, F., BALAN, B., RAYMOND, S. & CAMPBELL, J. 2016. Comparison of the effects of telephone suicide prevention help by volunteers and professional paid staff: results from studies in the USA and Quebec, Canada. *Suicide and Life-Threatening Behavior*, 46, 577–587.

MONTANA, P. G. 2017. Watch or report – livestream or help – Good Samaritan laws revisited: the need to create a duty to report. *Cleveland State Law Review*, 66, 533–558.

MÖRCH, C. M., CÔTÉ, L. P., CORTHÉSY-BLONDIN, L., PLOURDE-LÉVEILLÉ, L., DARGIS, L. & MISHARA, B. L. 2018. The Darknet and suicide. *Journal of Affective Disorders*, 241, 127–132.

MÖRCH, C. M., GUPTA, A. & MISHARA, B. L. 2020. Canada protocol: an ethical checklist for the use of artificial intelligence in suicide prevention and mental health. *Artificial Intelligence in Medicine*, 108.

MORDOR INTELLIGENCE INC. 2020. DTC (Direct to Consumer) DNA Test Kits Market – Growth, Trends, and Forecasts (2020-2025).

MORMONT, C. & WEISSTUB, D. N. 2020. Death and dying: from assisted suicide to COVID-19 and back. *Ethics, Medicine and Public Health*, 14, 100527.

MULDER, R., NEWTON-HOWES, G. & COID, J. W. 2016. The futility of risk prediction in psychiatry. *British Journal of Psychiatry*, 209, 271–272.

MURRAY, A. 2000. *Suicide in the Middle Ages: The Curse of Self-murder*. New York: Oxford University Press.

NAHME, P. E. & FELLER, Y. 2024. *Covenantal Thinking: Essays on the Philosophy and Theology of David Novak*. Toronto: University of Toronto Press.

NAITO, A. 2007. Internet suicide in Japan: implications for child and adolescent mental health. *Clinical Child Psychology and Psychiatry*, 12, 583–597.

NASHNOUSH, M. & SHEIKH, M. 2021. The morality of suicide. *Healthy Populations Journal*. https://doi.org/10.15273/hpj.v1i1.10589.

NATIONAL COMMISSION FOR THE PROTECTION OF HUMAN SUBJECTS OF BIOMEDICAL AND BEHAVIORAL RESEARCH 1979. *The Belmont Report*. https://www.hhs.gov/ohrp/regulations-and-policy/belmont-report/index.html.

NICOLINI, M., VANDENBERGHE, J. & GASTMANS, C. 2018. Substance use disorder and compulsory commitment to care: a care-ethical decision-making framework. *Scandinavian Journal of Caring Sciences*, 32, 1237–1246.

NICOLINI, M. E., KIM, S. Y. H., CHURCHILL, M. E. & GASTMANS, C. 2020. Should euthanasia and assisted suicide for psychiatric disorders be permitted? A systematic review of reasons. *Psychological Medicine*, 50, 1241–1256.

NIEDZWIEDZ, C., HAW, C., HAWTON, K. & PLATT, S. 2014. The definition and epidemiology of clusters of suicidal behavior: a systematic review. *Suicide and Life-Threatening Behavior*, 44, 569–581.

NORTHCUT, N. 2018. Is the Good Samaritan really good: a look into the possible harm caused by current Good Samaritan laws in response to biological epidemics. *Journal of Biosecurity, Biosafety and Biodefense Law*, 9, art. 20180002.

NUHN, A., HOLMES, S., KELLY, M., JUST, A., SHAW, J. & WIEBE, E. 2018. Experiences and perspectives of people who pursued medical assistance in dying: qualitative study in Vancouver, BC. *Canadian Family Physician*, 64, e380–e386.

OKAI, D., OWEN, G., MCGUIRE, H., SINGH, S., CHURCHILL, R. & HOTOPF, M. 2007. Mental capacity in psychiatric patients: systematic review. *British Journal of Psychiatry*, 191, 291–297.

OLSEN, D. P. 1998. Toward an ethical standard for coerced mental health treatment: least restrictive or most therapeutic? *Journal of Clinical Ethics*, 9, 235–246.

OLSEN, D. P. 2003. Influence and coercion: relational and rights-based ethical approaches to forced psychiatric treatment. *Journal of Psychiatric and Mental Health Nursing*, 10, 705–712.

ONWUTEAKA-PHILIPSEN, B. D., BRINKMAN-STOPPELENBURG, A., GWEN, C. P., DE JONG-KRUL, J. F. , VAN DELDEN, J. J. M. & VAN DER HEIDE, A. 2012. Trends in end-of-life practices before and after the enactment of the euthanasia law in the Netherlands from 1990 to 2010: a repeated cross-sectional survey. *The Lancet*, 380, 908–915.

O'REILLY, R. L. & GRAY, J. E. 2014. Canada's mental health legislation. *International Psychiatry*, 11, 65–67.

OWENS, D., HORROCKS, J. & HOUSE, A. 2002. Fatal and non-fatal repetition of self-harm: systematic review. *British Journal of Psychiatry*, 181, 193–199.

PACKMAN, W. L. & HARRIS, E. A. 1998. *Legal Issues and Risk Management in Suicidal Patients*. New York: Guilford Press.

PAUL, E., MERGL, R. & HEGERL, U. 2017. Has information on suicide methods provided via the internet negatively impacted suicide rates? *PLoS ONE*, 12, e0190136.

PERLIN, M. L., CUCOLO, H. E. & LYNCH, A. J. 2017. *Mental Disability Law: Cases and Materials, 3rd edition*. https://digitalcommons.nyls.edu/fac_books/39.

PERLS, A. 1911. Der Selbstmord nach der Halacha. *Monatsschrift fur Geschichte and Wissenschaft des Judentums*, 55, 287–295.

PHILLIPS, D. P. 1974. The influence of suggestion on suicide: substantive and theoretical implications of the Werther effect. *American Sociological Review*, 39, 340–354.

PHILLIPS, J. G., DIESFELD, K. & MANN, L. 2019. Instances of online suicide, the law and potential solutions. *Psychiatry, Psychology and Law*, 26, 423–440.

PILKINGTON, E. 2011. Outcry in America as pregnant women who lose babies face murder charges. *The Guardian*, 24 June.

PIRKIS, J. 2019. *Suicide and the Entertainment Media: A Critical Review*. https://mindframemedia.imgix.net/assets/src/uploads/Critical-Review-Suicide-and-the-entertainment-media.pdf.

PIRKIS, J., NEAL, L., DARE, A., BLOOD, R. W. & STUDDERT, D. 2009. Legal bans on pro-suicide web sites: an early retrospective from Australia. *Suicide and Life-Threatening Behavior*, 39, 190–193.

PIRKIS, J., BLOOD, R. W., KOSLOW, S. H., RUIZ, P. & NEMEROFF, C. B. 2014. Suicide and the media. In Koslow, S. H., Ruiz, P. & Nemeroff, C. B. (eds.), *A Concise Guide to Understanding Suicide: Epidemiology, Pathophysiology and Prevention*. Cambridge: Cambridge University Press.

PIRKIS, J., ROSSETTO, A., NICHOLAS, A., FTANOU, M., ROBINSON, J. & REAVLEY, N. 2017. Suicide prevention media campaigns: a systematic literature review. *Health Communication*. DOI: 10.1080/10410236.2017.1405484.

PITINI, E., DE VITO, C., MARZUILLO, C., D'ANDREA, E., ROSSO, A. , FEDERICI, A., DI MARIA, E. & VILLARI, P. 2018. How is genetic testing evaluated? A systematic review of the literature. *European Journal of Human Genetics*, 26, 605–615.

PLAISANCE, A., MISHARA, B. L., MASELLA, J., BRAVO, G., COUTURE, V. & TAPP, D. 2022. Quebec population highly supportive of extending Medical Aid in Dying to incapacitated persons and people suffering only from a mental illness: content analysis of attitudes and representations. *Ethics, Medicine and Public Health*, 21, 100759.

PLATO 1934. London: Dent & Sons. [Original work published BCE.]

POST, J., SPRINZAK, E. & DENNY, L. 2003. The terrorists in their own words: interviews with 35 incarcerated Middle Eastern terrorists. *Terrorism and Political Violence*, 15, 171–184.

PRADO, C. G. 1998. *The Last Choice: Preemptive Suicide in Advanced Age*. Westport: Greenwood Press.

PRADO, C. G. 2008. *Choosing to Die: Elective Death and Multiculturalism*. New York: Cambridge University Press.

PREUSS, J. 1978. *Biblical and Talmudic Medicine*. New York: Sanhedrin Press.

PUBLIC HEALTH DIVISION & CENTER FOR HEALTH STATISTICS 2020. *Oregon Death with Dignity Act 2019 Data Summary*.

PUBLIC HEALTH DIVISION & CENTER FOR HEALTH STATISTICS 2022. *Oregon Death with Dignity Act 2021 Data Summary*.

QUINN, G., MAHLER, C. & DE SCHUTTER, O. 2021. *Mandates of the Special Rapporteur on the Rights of Persons with Disabilities; the Independent Expert on the Enjoyment of All Human Rights by Older Persons; and the Special Rapporteur on Extreme Poverty and Human Rights*. Geneva: United Nations.

RAJAGOPAL, S. 2004. Suicide pacts and the internet. *BMJ: British Medical Journal*, 329, 1298–1299.

REGALADO, A. 2014. Could a genetic test predict the risk for suicide? *MIT Technology Review*. https://www.technologyreview.com/2014/08/13/171800/could-a-genetic-test-predict-the-risk-for-suicide/.

REGIONAL EUTHANASIA REVIEW COMMITTEES 2020. *Annual Report 2019*.

REUTER 2004. Internet pourrait encourager les suicides collectifs. *Le devoir*, 6 December.

RICHARD, J., WERTH, J. L., JR. & ROGERS, J. R. 2000. Rational and assisted suicidal communication on the internet: case example and discussion of ethical and practice issues. *Ethics and Behavior*, 10, 215–238.

RICHMOND, C. 2005. Dame Cicely Saunders. *British Medical Journal*, 331, 238.

RIETJENS, J. A., VAN TOL, D. G., SCHERMER, M. & VAN DER HEIDE, A. 2009. Judgement of suffering in the case of a euthanasia request in the Netherlands. *Journal of Medical Ethics*, 35, 502–507.

RIMMER, A. 2019. Social media: suicide promotion and anti-vaccine content must be banned, says BMA. *British Medical Journal*, 365, l4425.

RIPKE, S., O'DUSHLAINE, C., CHAMBERT, K., MORAN, J. L., KÄHLER, A. K., AKTERIN, S., BERGEN, S. E., COLLINS, A. L., CROWLEY, J. J., FROMER, M., KIM, Y., LEE, S. H., MAGNUSSON, P. K., SANCHEZ, N., STAHL, E. A., WILLIAMS, S., WRAY, N. R., XIA, K., BETTELLA, F., BORGLUM, A. D., BULIK-SULLIVAN, B. K., CORMICAN, P., CRADDOCK, N., DE LEEUW, C., DURMISHI, N., GILL, M., GOLIMBET, V., HAMSHERE, M. L., HOLMANS, P., HOUGAARD, D. M., KENDLER, K. S., LIN, K., MORRIS, D. W., MORS, O., MORTENSEN, P. B., NEALE, B. M., O'NEILL, F. A., OWEN, M. J., MILOVANCEVIC, M. P., POSTHUMA, D., POWELL, J., RICHARDS, A. L., RILEY, B. P., RUDERFER, D., RUJESCU, D., SIGURDSSON, E., SILAGADZE, T., SMIT, A. B., STEFANSSON, H., STEINBERG, S., SUVISAARI, J., TOSATO, S., VERHAGE, M., WALTERS, J. T., LEVINSON, D. F., GEJMAN, P. V., KENDLER, K. S., LAURENT, C., MOWRY, B. J., O'DONOVAN, M. C., OWEN, M. J., PULVER, A. E., RILEY, B. P., SCHWAB, S. G., WILDENAUER, D. B., DUDBRIDGE, F., HOLMANS, P., SHI, J., ALBUS, M., ALEXANDER, M., CAMPION, D., COHEN, D., DIKEOS, D., DUAN, J., EICHHAMMER, P., GODARD, S., HANSEN, M., LERER, F. B., LIANG, K. Y., MAIER, W., MALLET, J., NERTNEY, D. A., NESTADT, G., NORTON, N., O'NEILL, F. A., PAPADIMITRIOU, G. N., RIBBLE, R., SANDERS, A. R., SILVERMAN, J. M., WALSH, D., WILLIAMS, N. M., WORMLEY, B., ARRANZ, M. J., BAKKER, S., BENDER, S., BRAMON, E., COLLIER, D., CRESPO-FACORRO, B., HALL, J., IYEGBE, C., et al. 2013. Genome-wide association analysis identifies 13 new risk loci for schizophrenia. *Nature Genetics*, 45, 1150–1159.

ROBSON, A., SCRUTTON, F., WILKINSON, L. & MACLEOD, F. 2010. The risk of suicide in cancer patients: a review of the literature. *Psycho-oncology*, 19, 1250–1258.

RUBINSTEIN, E. 2003. Going beyond parents and institutional review boards in protecting children involved in nontherapeutic research. *Golden Gate University Law Review*, 33, 251–294.

RUISSEN, A. M., WIDDERSHOVEN, G. A. M., MEYNEN, G., ABMA, T. A. & VAN BALKOM, A. J. L. M. 2012. A systematic review of the literature about competence and poor insight. *Acta Psychiatrica Scandinavica*, 125, 103–113.

RURUP, M. L., MULLER, M. T., ONWUTEAKA-PHILIPSEN, B. D., VAN DER HEIDE, A., VAN DER WAL, G. & VAN DER MAAS, P. J. 2005. Requests for euthanasia or physician-assisted suicide from older persons who do not have a severe disease: an interview study. *Psychological Medicine*, 35, 665–671.

RUSH, B. 1812. *Medical Inquiries and Observations, Upon the Diseases of the Mind*. Philadelphia: Kimber & Richardson. http://resource.nlm.nih .gov/2569037R.

SADZAGLISHVILI, S., GOTSIRIDZE, T. & LEKESHVILI, K. 2021. Ethical considerations for social work research with vulnerable children and their families. *Research on Social Work Practice*, 31, 351–359.

SAIGLE, V., SÉGUIN, M. & RACINE, E. 2017. Identifying gaps in suicide research: a scoping review of ethical challenges and proposed recommendations. *IRB Ethics & Human Research*, 39, 1–9.

SAMARITANS 2020. Samaritans Annual Report and Account 2019–2020. https://media.samaritans.org/documents/Samaritans-Annual-Report-Accounts-2019-2020.pdf.

SAREEN, J., HENRIKSEN, C. A., STEIN, M. B., AFIFI, T. O., LIX, L. M. & ENNS, M. W. 2013. Common mental disorder diagnosis and need for treatment are not the same: findings from a population-based longitudinal survey. *Psychological Medicine*, 43, 1941–1951.

SAVULESCU, J. 1994. Rational desires and the limitation of life-sustaining treatment. *Bioethics*, 8, 191–222.

SAYA, A., BRUGNOLI, C., PIAZZI, G., LIBERATO, D., CIACCIA, G. D., NIOLU, C. & SIRACUSANO, A. 2019. Criteria, procedures, and future prospects of involuntary treatment in psychiatry around the world: a narrative review. *Frontiers in Psychiatry*, 10. https://doi.org/10.3389/fpsyt.2019.00271.

SCHARRER, E. 2015. The behavioral, affective, and cognitive implications of media violence: complex relationships between young people and texts. In LEMISH, D. (ed.) *The Routledge International Handbook of Children, Adolescents and Media*. New York: Routledge.

SCHIZOPHRENIA PSYCHIATRIC GENOME-WIDE ASSOCIATION STUDY (GWAS) CONSORTIUM 2011. Genome-wide association study identifies five new schizophrenia loci. *Nature Genetics*, 43, 969–978.

SCHIZOPHRENIA WORKING GROUP OF THE PSYCHIATRIC GENOMICS CONSORTIUM 2014. Biological insights from 108 schizophrenia-associated genetic loci. *Nature*, 511, 421–427.

SCHNABEL, P., MEYBOOM-DE JONG, B., SCHUDEL, W. J., CLEIREN, C. P. M., MEVIS, P. A. M., VERKERK, M. J., HEIDE, A. V. D. & HESSELMANN, G. 2016. *Voltooid Leven: Over Hulp Bij Zelfdoding van Mensen Die Hun Leven Voltooid Achten [Completed Life: On Assisted Suicide in People Who Consider Their Life Completed]*. Leiden: Leiden University.

SCORDATO, M. R. 2008. Understanding the absence of a duty to reasonably rescue in American tort law. *Tulane Law Review*, 82, 1447–1504.

SCOTT, A. 2011. *Talking to the Enemy: Religion, Brotherhood, and the (Un) Making of Terrorists*. London: Harper Collins e-books.

SEGAL, S. P., HAYES, S. L. & RIMES, L. 2017. The utility of outpatient commitment: I. A need for treatment and a least restrictive alternative to psychiatric hospitalization. *Psychiatric Services*, 68, 1247–1254.

SENATE OF CANADA 1995. *Of Life and Death – Final Report*. Ottawa: Special Senate Committee on Euthanasia and Assisted Suicide, Senate of Canada.

SHAPIRO, D. 1965. *Neurotic Styles*. New York: BasicBooks.

SHNEIDMAN, E. S. 1973. *On the Nature of Suicide*. San Francisco: Jossey-Bass.

SHULTZINER, D. 2007. Human dignity: functions and meanings. In MALPAS, J. & LICKISS, N. (eds.) *Perspectives on Human Dignity: A Conversation*. Dordrecht: Springer.

SINGARAVELU, V., STEWART, A., ADAMS, J., SIMKIN, S. & HAWTON, K. 2015. Information-seeking on the internet. *Crisis*, 36, 211–219.

SKLAR, R. B. 2011. The capable mental health patient's right to refuse treatment special section: towards autonomy: exploring the clinical, legal and ethical aspects of mental capacity. *McGill Journal of Law and Health*, 5, 291.

SMETS, T., COHEN, J., BILSEN, J., VAN WESEMAEL, Y., RURUP, M. L. & DELIENS, L. 2012. The labelling and reporting of euthanasia by Belgian physicians: a study of hypothetical cases. *European Journal of Public Health*, 22, 19–26.

SMITH, G. J. H. 2002. *Internet Law and Regulation*. London: Sweet & Maxwell.

SPECIAL JOINT COMMITTEE ON MEDICAL ASSISTANCE IN DYING 2023. *Medical Assistance in Dying in Canada: Choices for Canadians*. https://www.parl.ca/Content/Committee/441/AMAD/Reports/RP12234766/amadrp02/amadrp02-e.pdf.

SPOLETINI, I., GIANNI, W., CALTAGIRONE, C., MADAIO, R., REPETTO, L. & SPALLETTA, G. 2011. Suicide and cancer: where do we go from here? *Critical Reviews in Oncology and Hematology*, 78, 206–219.

STACK, S. 2003. Media coverage as a risk factor in suicide. *Journal of Epidemiology and Community Health*, 57, 238–240.

STACK, S. 2005. Suicide in the media: a quantitative review of studies based on nonfictional stories. *Suicide and Life-Threatening Behavior*, 35, 121–133.

STACK, S. & KPOSOWA, A. J. 2016. Culture and suicide acceptability: a cross-national, multilevel analysis. *Sociological Quarterly*, 57, 282–303.

STARCK, C. 2002. The religious and philosophical background of human dignity and its place in modern constitutions. In KRETZMER, D. & KLEIN, E. (eds.) *The Concept of Human Dignity in Human Rights Discourse*. London: The Hague.

STOJANOVIĆ, G. 2020. The ethical legacy of Hippocrates. *Scripta Medica*, 51, 275–283.

STONE, A. A. & STROMBERG, C. D. 1976. *Mental Health and Law: A System in Transition*. New York: J. Aronson.

STROMBERG, C. D. & STONE, A. A. 1983. A model state law on civil commitment of the mentally ill. *Harvard Journal of Legislation*, 20, 275–396.

SUDOL, K. & MANN, J. J. 2017. Biomarkers of suicide attempt behavior: towards a biological model of risk. *Current Psychiatry Reports*, 19, 31.

SVEEN, C. A. & WALBY, F. A. 2008. Suicide survivors' mental health and grief reactions: a systematic review of controlled studies. *Suicide and Life-Threatening Behavior*, 38, 13–29.

SWANSON, J. W., SWARTZ, M. S. & MOSELEY, D. D. 2017. US outpatient commitment in context: when is it ethical and how can we tell? In Buchanan, A. & Wootton, L. (eds.) *Care of the Mentally Disordered Offender in the Community*, 2nd edition. New York: Oxford University Press.

SWICK. 2005. *Platform for Internet Content Selection (PICS) Platform for Internet Content Selection (PICS)* [Online]. W3C. Available: http://www.w3.org/PICS/ [Accessed 14 September 2023]. Internet Archive. [http://web.archive.org/web/20041009202820/http://www.robirda.com/cancare.html].

SZASZ, T. 1986. The case against suicide prevention. *American Psychologist*, 41, 806–812.

SZMUKLER, G. & HOLLOWAY, F. 1998. Mental health legislation is now a harmful anachronism. *Psychiatric Bulletin*, 22, 662–665.

TANAKA, H., TSUKUMA, H., MASAOKA, T., AJIKI, W., KOYAMA, Y., KINOSHITA, N., HASUO, S. & OSHIMA, A. 1999. Suicide risk among cancer patients: experience at one medical center in Japan, 1978–1994. *Japanese Journal of Cancer Research*, 90, 812–817.

TAYLOR, D. H., JR., OSTERMANN, J., VAN HOUTVEN, C. H., TULSKY, J. A. & STEINHAUSER, K. 2007. What length of hospice use maximizes reduction in medical expenditures near death in the US Medicare program? *Social Science and Medicine*, 65, 1466–1478.

TAYLOR, S. 2019. Kill me through the phone: the legality of encouraging suicide in an increasingly digital world. *Brigham Young University Law Review*, 613 (2020).

TEUTSCH, S. M., BRADLEY, L. A., PALOMAKI, G. E., HADDOW, J. E., PIPER, M., CALONGE, N., DOTSON, W. D., DOUGLAS, M. P. & BERG, A. O. 2009. The Evaluation of Genomic Applications in Practice and Prevention (EGAPP) initiative: methods of the EGAPP Working Group. *Genetics in Medicine*, 11, 3–14.

THE AMERICAN ASSOCIATION OF SUICIDOLOGY. 2017. *Statement of the American Association of Suicidology: suicide is not the same as physician aid in dying* [Online]. Available: https://suicidology.org/wp-content/uploads/2019/07/AAS-PAD-Statement-Approved-10.30.17-ed-10-30-17.pdf [Accessed 14 September 2023]._Internet Archive_. [http://web.archive.org/web/20210801113601/https://suicidology.org/wp-content/uploads/2019/07/AAS-PAD-Statement-Approved-10.30.17-ed-10-30-17.pdf]

THE HALIFAX GROUP 2020. *MAiD Legislation at a Crossroads: Persons with Mental Disorders as Their Sole Underlying Medical Condition*. Montreal: Institute for Research on Public Policy.

THE MINISTRY OF LAW AND JUSTICE 2017. *The Mental Healthcare Act. 04/0007/2003–17*. The Gazette of India.

THOMASMA, D. C. & WEISSTUB, D. N. 2004. *The Variables of Moral Capacity*. Dordrecht: Kluwer Academic Publishers.

TIDEMALM, D., RUNESON, B., WAERN, M., FRISELL, T., CARLSTRÖM, E., LICHTENSTEIN, P. & LÅNGSTRÖM, N. 2011. Familial clustering of suicide risk: a total population study of 11.4 million individuals. *Psychological Medicine*, 41, 2527–2534.

TONG, R. 2000. Duty to die. In HUMBER, J. M. & ALMEDER, R. F. (eds.) *Is There a Duty to Die?* Totowa: Humana Press.

TORREY, E. F. & ZDANOWICZ, M. 2001. Outpatient commitment: what, why, and for whom. *Psychiatric Services*, 52, 337–341.

TOTARO, S., TOFFOL, E. & SCOCCO, P. 2016. Suicide prevention and the internet, risks and opportunities: a narrative review. *Suicidology Online*, 7, 63–73.

TOWNSEND, E. 2007. Suicide terrorists: are they suicidal? *Suicide and Life-Threatening Behavior*, 37, 35–49.

TUCKER, R. P., TACKETT, M. J., GLICKMAN, D. & REGER, M. A. 2019. Ethical and practical considerations in the use of a predictive model to trigger suicide prevention interventions in healthcare settings. *Suicide and Life-Threatening Behavior*, 49, 382–392.

TUNG, J., DECARIA, K., DUDGEON, D., GREEN, E., MOXAM, R. S., NIU, J. & RAHAL, R. 2018. Acute-care hospital use patterns near end-of-life for cancer patients who die in hospital in Canada. *Journal of Global Oncology*, 4, 109s.

TURECKI, G., BRENT, D. A., GUNNELL, D., O'CONNOR, R. C., OQUENDO, M. A., PIRKIS, J. & STANLEY, B. H. 2019. Suicide and suicide risk. *Nature Reviews Disease Primers*, 5, 74.

TURKHEIMER, E. 2000. Three laws of behavior genetics and what they mean. *Current Directions in Psychological Science*, 9, 160–164.

TUSIEWICZ, K., WACHEŁKO, O., ZAWADZKI, M., CHŁOPAŚ-KONOWAŁEK, A., JUREK, T., KAWECKI, J. & SZPOT, P. 2022. The dark side of social media: two deaths related with chloroform intoxication. *Journal of Forensic Sciences*, 67, 1300–1307.

TWOHEY, M. & DANCE, G. X. J. 2021. Where the despairing log on, and learn ways to die. *The New York Times*, 9 December.

UELMEN, A. J. 2016. Where morality and the law coincide: how legal obligations of bystanders may be informed by the social teachings of Pope Francis. *Seattle University Law Review*, 40, 1359.

UN GENERAL ASSEMBLY 1966. International Covenant on Civil and Political Rights. Resolution 2200A (XXI). *United Nations, Treaty Series*, 999, 171.

UNITED NATIONS. 2006. *Convention of the Rights of Persons with Disabilities.* New York: United Nations.

UNITED NATIONS HUMAN RIGHTS COUNCIL 2019. *General Assembly Official Records Seventy-fourth Session Supplement No. 53 A (A/74/53/Add.1).* New York: United Nations.

UNITED NATIONS HUMAN RIGHTS COMMITTEE (HRC) 2019. *International Covenant on Civil and Political Rights, General comment no. 36, Article 6 (Right to Life).* New York: United Nations.

VAN HEERINGEN, K. & MANN, J. J. 2014. The neurobiology of suicide. *Lancet Psychiatry*, 1, 63–72.

VERHOFSTADT, M., THIENPONT, L. & PETERS, G. J. Y. 2017. When unbearable suffering incites psychiatric patients to request euthanasia: qualitative study. *British Journal of Psychiatry*, 211, 238–245.

VOLOKH, E. 1999. Duties to rescue and the anticooperative effects of law essay. *The Georgetown Law Journal*, 88, 105.

VULNERABLE PERSONS SECRETARIAT 2020. *Voices from the Margins.* The Vulnerable Persons Standard. https://static1.squarespace.com/static/56bb84cb01dbae77f988b71a/t/5f9065e56d65272858143fca/16032.

WEBSTER 1966. *Webster's New World Dictionary of the American Language.* New York: World Publishing Company.

WEINER, J. 2022. *Care and Covenant: A Jewish Bioethic of Responsibility.* Washington, DC: Georgetown University Press.

WEINRIB, E. J. 1980. The case for a duty to rescue. *Yale Law Journal,* 90, 247–293.

WEISSTUB, D. N. 1990. *Enquiry on Mental Competency: Final Report.* Toronto: Ontario Ministry of Health.

WEISSTUB, D. N. 1998. The ethical parameters of experimentation. In WEISSTUB, D. N. (ed.) *Research on Human Subjects: Ethics, Law and Public Policy.* Oxford: Pergamon Press.

WEISSTUB, D. N. 2001. *Les populations vulnérables.* Paris: L'Harmattan.

WEISSTUB, D. N. & PINTOS, G. D. A. 2008. *Autonomy and Human Rights in Health Care: An International Perspective.* Dordrecht: Springer.

WEISSTUB, D. N. & THOMASMA, D. C. 2001. Human dignity, vulnerability, personhood. In WEISSTUB, D. N. & THOMASMA, D. C. (eds.) *Personhood and Health Care.* Dordrecht: Springer.

WERTH, J. L., JR. 2001. U.S. involuntary mental health commitment statutes: requirements for persons perceived to be a potential harm to self. *Suicide and Life-Threatening Behavior,* 31, 348–357.

WETTSTEIN, R. 2003. Specific issues in psychiatric malpractice. In ROSNER, R. (ed.) *Principles and Practice of Forensic Psychiatry,* 2nd edition. Baco Raton: CRC Press.

WHITEFORD, H. A., HARRIS, M. G., MCKEON, G., BAXTER, A., PENNELL, C., BARENDREGT, J. J. & WANG, J. 2013. Estimating remission from untreated major depression: a systematic review and meta-analysis. *Psychological Medicine,* 43, 1569–1585.

WORLD HEALTH ORGANIZATION 2014. *Preventing Suicide: A Global Imperative.* Geneva: World Health Organization.

WORLD HEALTH ORGANIZATION. 2021a. *Suicide* [Online]. Geneva: World Health Organization. Available at: https://www.who.int/news-room/fact-sheets/detail/suicide.

WORLD HEALTH ORGANIZATION. 2021b. Suicide worldwide in 2019: global health estimates. https://apps.who.int/iris/bitstream/handle/10665/341728/9789240026643-eng.pdf.

WRIGHT, C. F. & KROESE, M. 2010. Evaluation of genetic tests for susceptibility to common complex diseases: why, when and how? *Human Genetics*, 127, 125–134.

YAREMKO, O. & BANAKH, S. 2018. Incitement to suicide with social networks and the internet: problems of criminal liability in Ukraine. *ACIT 2018*. Czech Republic.

ZIMBROFF, R. M., ORNSTEIN, K. A. & SHEEHAN, O. C. 2021. Home-based primary care: a systematic review of the literature, 2010–2020. *Journal of the American Geriatrics Society*, 69, 2963–2972.

Index

Printed in the United States
by Baker & Taylor Publisher Services